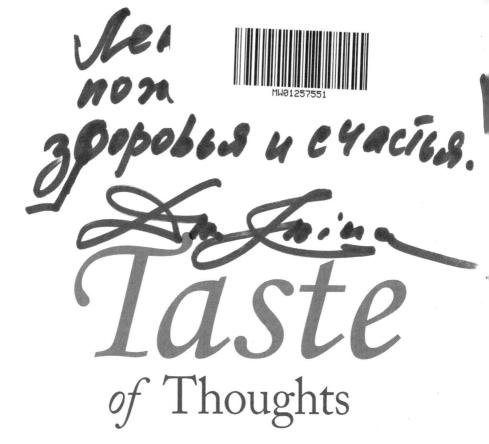

Taste

of Thoughts

Improve Your Health and Whole Life

Dr. Irina Koles

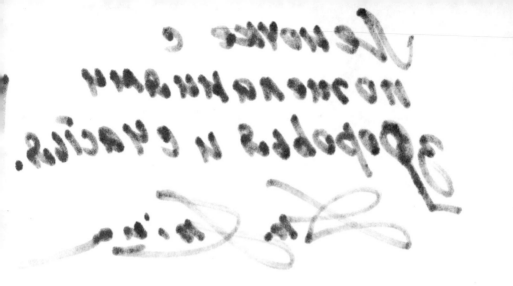

ISBN-10: 1468035770
ISBN-13: 9781468035773

Table of Contents

Introduction

*T*he obesity problem in the US is now a reality, not a possibility. It is estimated that 34% of adults and 17% of children and adolescents are obese. Obesity is responsible for a number of diseases, even death, and costs individuals and the healthcare system millions of dollars.

At the same time, dozens of diets and nutrition plans are readily available. Every weekly magazine offers new information about dieting. In addition, the manufacturers produce more and more healthy food. So, what happens? Why, in spite of the availability of so much information and a wide choice of healthy food, people are still overweight and obese?

Don't we know what we should do? Don't we know that an apple is healthier than a donut? Sure we do! We KNOW that we eat wrong. We all are aware of different diets, healthy nutrition plans and fitness centers. We certainly know WHAT is wrong and WHAT we should do; we just don't know HOW to do that.

* HOW to uncover the deep roots of extra pounds

* HOW to overcome the unhealthy habits

* HOW to overcome the obstacles

* HOW to set the right goals

* HOW to develop healthy habits

* HOW not to get lost among a huge choice of food

* HOW to transform a diet to a healthy lifestyle

* HOW to make a right choice on an everyday basis

* HOW to make a right choice in restaurants or social events

* HOW to make it easy

* HOW to keep the desired healthy weight forever

Constantly, so many people are struggling with their extra pounds. For months and even years, they follow different diets and vigorously exercise. In some cases, this behavior helps many of us successfully reach our desired weight. However, only 10% of people are able to keep that weight for more than one year. Think about that statistic. After all that struggling, nine out of ten people will be back to their previous weight in less than only ONE YEAR! If the statistics were the opposite and only one person out of ten could not keep his/her weight, we would probably attribute it to the individual's weak personality and irresponsibility. But, could nine out of ten really be weak and irresponsible people? It sounds unbelievable. Why can't people keep what they have already achieved?

The answer is simple. No diet can last forever. It is almost impossible to follow a plan during one's entire life. When the plan is over — the weight is back. The problem needs to be addressed on a much deeper level: first in your mind, then on your plate.

This book will teach you HOW to do that and will answer all the other HOWs.

* You will understand what actually happens in your body when you eat

* You will discover that we gain weight not because we eat too much, but because we have unhealthy eating habits

* You will look at yourself and at your childhood and will find out the real reasons for your current extra pounds

* You will discover your Eating Blueprint and how to change it in your favor

* You will know how to recognize unhealthy thoughts and how to replace them with beneficial ones

* You will develop a healthy Eating Blueprint

* You will stop counting calories and being afraid of eating some extra food. Food is not your enemy; it will become your friend

* You will learn how to make the right choice out of a vast array of food on an everyday basis

* You will enjoy social, family and professional events without depriving yourself of the pleasure of cooking and eating

* You will experience feelings of physical and emotional energy, along with a clear understanding of why this happens to you

* You will invest in your health, and prevent the many diseases that can be caused by being overweight

* Your new health and vitality path will help you improve your personal and professional life

* You will use simple and healthy cooking recipes and learn how to adjust your own favorite recipes

* Once you adopt a new way of thinking and eating, it will become your lifestyle and will last forever

Enjoy Your Journey to Your Healthy and Happy Life!

෴

Dedication

*T*his book is dedicated to the man of my life, the most loving and supportive person, my mentor and my coach — my son Roman.

He is the one who 'dragged' me into the Personal Development world (OK, I admit that he's got some genes) and supported me through all our life challenges. He was the first person with whom I shared my business idea. He helped me to stay focused on my dream and make it a reality.

You are the best thing that has ever happened to me!

THANK YOU!

Acknowledgements

*F*irst, I am sincerely grateful to my parents Adolf and Roza, for their unconditional love and support, their understanding, forgiveness and patience, especially when I was so busy writing this book and developing my business. We are very close, and it was very hard not to see each other during that time.

Also, thanks to my lovely son Roman. He supported me, coached me and led me through the challenges. He constantly inspired me, and convinced me to believe in myself.

Special thanks to Steve Harrison and his coaching team. Without your help, this book would never exist. When I came to your program, I knew absolutely nothing about writing a book, and even less about publicity and marketing. From the very first seminar in Philadelphia, I understood that I was in the right place, at the right time and I was ready to learn. You taught me those strategies, and became a great personal and business model for me. Thank you all, from the bottom of my heart.

Thank you, all my Personal Development gurus: Jack Canfield, Joe Vitale, Anthony Robbins, T. Harv Eker, Brian Tracy, James Arthur Ray, John Grey, Dr.Wayne Dyer, Jim Rohn, Mike Dooley, Bob Proctor, Susan Jeffers, Robin Sharma, Paulo Coelho, John C. Maxwell, Robert Kyosaki, and of course to Dale Carnegie, Napoleon Hill, Jose Silva, David J. Schwartz and many others. If you only knew what impact you've had on my life! Without you, I would never have become the person I am now, and I would never be where I now am. Thank you for being a huge part of my life.

Thanks to French nutrition and culinary guru Michel Montignac. His books about Low Glycemic Index nutrition changed my Eating Blueprint and my whole life. I am sorry it is too late to express my appreciation and thank you in person.

To my friends in the US, Israel and Russia who always believed in me and inspired me, gave me some great ideas and helped me to stay on track, I thank you all.

Most of all, I would like to thank God for my health, optimistic character, strength, vision and purpose. Thank you for helping me to persevere through the struggles and the difficulties. Thank you for blessing me with strong willpower and the ability to believe in success despite tough circumstances. Thank you for keeping me motivated in spite of my age, loneliness, immigrant status, a language barrier and low budget. Thanks for giving me the courage to proceed on blind faith and do whatever was necessary on my journey towards success.

THANK YOU

Preface

My Dear Reader,

Maybe you accidentally found my book, while browsing the shelves filled with books on sports, politics and sex. Maybe you're even thinking, "What? Another book about dieting? No way!"

Calm down. In fact, it's just the opposite. This book is about NOT dieting. It is about enjoying your life, social events and cooking (if you enjoy doing so), while maintaining a healthy eating lifestyle and vitality. This book explains how to taste your thoughts before tasting food on your plate. Your weight does not matter. If you are only a little overweight, not dramatically overweight or obese, this book will help you understand what happens in your body when you eat, as well as show you how to eat healthier and keep your desired weight forever.

The information in this book comes from a retired physician who is now a professional health coach. I'm passionate about what I do, and will present my advice and approach in a way that is easy and fun for you to understand.

In a good way, my life has been very challenging. I went through two immigrations, twice starting life from scratch and absorbing two absolutely different cultures. I changed apartments, cities and countries, learned two new languages, then found myself divorced after 21 years of marriage, changed jobs and even my profession. Along the way, I had to make many other life-changing decisions. I am grateful for those challenges because they made me the person who I am today.

Growing up in Russia, I had a happy childhood. Both my parents are University professors; education was always a priority in our family. We were not rich or famous, but we had enough money for everyday needs. I was happy with what I had, but I always desired more, and kept my expectations high.

All my life, I was interested in Personal Development topics. I have read many books by great people such as John Maxwell, Dale Carnegie, Napoleon Hill, Jack Canfield, Anthony Robbins, and other brilliant authors of the New Age movement. I listened to as many audiotapes as I could find, and attended dozens of seminars. Learning about self-improvement has made an impact on my life. It has made me stronger and fortified my character.

I graduated from medical school and worked as a physician. At the age of 28, with my husband and our 5 year old son, I emigrated from Russia. We left our jobs, parents, relatives and friends and moved to Israel, where we knew no one, and had nothing. We started our life literally from ground zero. We went through the first Gulf war in 1990, and lived under the stressful ongoing Middle East conflicts.

We accomplished a great deal over the next 13 years. We both practiced medicine and were finally living a comfortable life. This is where I won the Green Card lottery and had a tough decision to face. By that time, we were not 28 but 41, and had to decide if we wanted to leave everything behind (again!) and move to the United States to build our life from scratch (again!). It was a tough decision. However, in my opinion, nothing is worse than missing an opportunity that could change your life forever. We couldn't afford to miss this chance, so we took the risk.

The first few years in the U.S. were very difficult. After being a doctor for years, I found myself working in retail stores 12 hours a day. My husband at the time was going through the processing of getting board certified, and our son was going to a new high school. It was a hard time, but I didn't regret our choice. I applied to college and got a Master's Degree in Healthcare Management. The new analytical job in the hospital was extremely complex, but brought me many interesting experiences and new skills. Risk and challenges only make us stronger. As of now, I am so happy and grateful to live in the U.S., and have new friends, new life and most of all — my own business!

After studying the topics of Self Development and Healthy Lifestyle for years, one day I realized that I should combine them! The entire puzzle just came together and the idea of 'Journey to YOUR Destiny' was born.

By age 30, I had never used any diets. I love to cook, and I always threw parties for 20 to 30 people - and I cooked all the food by myself. I enjoyed all of that without even thinking about any extra pounds. But, after age 30, I started to gain weight. I definitely did not like that, and began practicing a low-calorie diet like many other people. I lost my extra pounds successfully, and periodically allowed myself to eat whatever I wanted at parties or restaurants. Initially, this strategy worked well, but then something strange happened; I did not eat much, but I was gaining weight. So, I started to eat even less, practiced some magic by taking "herbal" weight loss pills, but I still gained weight. It was depressing and stressful.

One day, I found a book by Michel Montignac *Eat Yourself Slim* and discovered a system based on something called a "Glycemic Index." I read the book, found it interesting, but totally...odd. However, something about that book forced me to consider an unusual approach to nutrition. I had to re-read the book three times and it took me about two months to change my perception, to accept a new theory and to start practicing that. I was now THINKING differently and the results were amazing! I could eat the food that I had not had for years! It even became an interesting journey; I enjoyed discovering new products and could easily adjust my favorite recipes. It was like a dream come true. I ate, I cooked and I stayed slim and energetic!

I have been following that system since then, and still have joy and real passion for it. I've taught it to hundreds of my patients, my family, friends, and everyone who is interested in keeping the ideal weight, being healthy and enjoy life.

However, being overweight is not just a nutrition issue. It's a problem involving nutritional, behavioral and family habits, lack of self-esteem, miscorrelation between willpower and imagination, feelings of guilt and judgment. It cannot be treated with just any low-calorie diet and hardcore exercises. It should be treated as a whole-body problem with a complex approach. The focus should be on the person, not on the symptom. When you change the roots, you'll change the fruits.

To your Health and Success,

Dr.Irina

Chapter 1 : Personal Blueprint

"Life is your imagination, not your history"
Stephen Covey

W hat is a Blueprint? This is how it is described in the dictionary:

Blueprint:

1: *a photographic print in white on a bright blue ground or blue on a white ground used especially for copying maps, mechanical drawings, and architects' plans*

2: *something resembling a blueprint (as in serving as a model or providing guidance); especially: a detailed plan or program*

For example, a house blueprint is a detailed plan or design for that particular building. It is created BEFORE the house physically built.

The same applies to our personal blueprint. There is a particular design, a plan, an existed programming in our mind, which determines our behavior and our physical word.

Where it is coming from and how it existed? First, heredity. Genetic information from our parents and grandparents makes us unique. Then, during the embryo stage, we are influenced by our mother's habits, behavior and lifestyle. Therefore, at birth, each of us already has some character traits. Some babies are quieter, other more active, sleepy or not, crying and sad, or smiling and curious. Each baby is a composite of original physiological, psychological and mental patterns. What the baby doesn't yet have is his or her own knowledge and experience. Babies cannot survive without support and external care.

Now, after being comfortable and secure in a mother's womb, we find ourselves outside growing, and learning life by ourselves. We learn from our parents, other relatives, friends, teachers, religious leaders, as well as from culture, media and society. This influence is very strong during the early years of our life, when these forces literally 'paint' our blueprint hour after hour, day after day. Very soon each of us has a personal blueprint embedded in our subconscious mind, and that blueprint more than anything else determines our life behavior. Actually, we have many different blueprints: for personal behavior, for education, money, love and relationships, for our eating habits and general health, self-image and self-esteem, for our emotions, spirit and life in general.

Is our blueprint very strong and one that will last forever? That's a difficult question. Imagine a mansion, which was built 150 years ago and still has the same design and structure. It is strong and established; it is not easy to change. However, can it be rebuilt? Absolutely! Should we start rebuilding it from the roof, or paint its walls first? I don't think so... To get a new mansion, the changes should be made in its original plan, in that 150 year old mansion blueprint! Then, according to the new blueprint, it will be rebuilt and become a new gorgeous mansion!

The same applies to people. We can live our life and be happy with that (or not) without changing anything for years. Then something happens, and we feel the desperate desire for rebuilding. We are ready for remodeling and renovation. The good news is that in our case, we don't need to wait until someone comes to change our original blueprint. It's possible, though, and perhaps fortunate if a person or several people will influence our existed blueprint positively by installing better files. But what if they don't? What if they rebuild it as a country style, when over your entire life you were dreaming about contemporary? It happens, right? If you do not manage your life by yourself, someone else will, and not always in your favor. Then, you'll live the life of his/her/their dreams, not yours. Is this what you want to happen? I hope not. We can and should do it by ourselves. Changing your life blueprint in YOUR favor is YOUR privilege. You should aim to act by yourself according to YOUR desires, YOUR wishes, YOUR goals and YOUR dreams.

Seriously, who knows your dreams better than YOU?

Eating Blueprint

Let's admit it, we LOVE to eat. At least I do, for sure. We eat not because we just need a refill; we eat because we enjoy it. Nowadays, the variety of food products is huge and renewed endlessly. There are so many choices that I think we hardly have the time to taste even a fraction of the offerings in supermarkets. We all have our everyday preferences, plus we periodically buy new food according to a recipe or recent commercial.

We may not be conscious of it, but our preferences are dictated by our Eating Blueprint. Have you ever looked at other people's shopping carts at the supermarket? It is interesting to see how differently people buy their food. Some shopping carts are full with pre-cooked packages, others with snacks, some overloaded with cookies, bagels, ice cream and waffles; you can also recognize fish lovers, meat lovers or vegetarians. Where those preferences are coming from? They come from people's Eating Blueprints.

Once I was at the farmers market with my friend who has three children. I was shocked when she started to throw huge packages of different candies into her cart. She was getting pounds and pounds of Twix, Snickers, M&Ms and Hershey's Bars. Since we are very good friends, I didn't hesitate to stop her and ask why she was buying so many sweets. Her response: "The kids LOVE them, and they're much cheaper here!" "But farmers are selling super fresh fruits and berries!" I replied. "You'd better buy THEM for your kids!

They would love whatever you bring home!" Surprisingly, she began following my advice, took away all those candies and bought strawberries, peaches, mangos and even black and red currants. A little later, we finished our shopping and drove home. She got home before I did, and by the time I reached my home, my phone was ringing. She said excitedly, "I can't believe it! The kids LOVE fruits and berries! They are SO happy and didn't even ask for the candies they wanted me to buy!" There you go. Kids will love whatever you feed them from early childhood. If your house is full of candies and cookies, they are getting a "candy-cookie" blueprint. If you buy and cook healthy food, they are getting "fruit-vegetables-meat-fish-grains" blueprint, which is without a doubt, much healthier.

Have you ever thought of YOUR Eating Blueprint?

It doesn't matter if you overweight or not. You may be at your ideal weight, or four pounds less, or 50 pounds more. This book is not about numbers. It is about YOU, about your FEELINGS toward those numbers and most importantly, about your health.

The Truth about Calories

"To be successful, all you have to do is give up everything you know."

Asara Lovejoy

Counting calories has become an epidemic. There is no food without calories listed, and in many restaurants, you can see the amount of calories consumed with every dish. They are listed with suspicious accuracy. You never see numbers like 250 or 400; it is usually 249 and 253, or 397 and 401. What is it all about? What is the meaning of the term calorie? Here is the definition:

*A **calorie** is the amount of energy needed to raise the temperature of one gram of water for one degree of centigrade.*

The human body needs energy for:

* Maintaining a body temperature at 98.6° F
* Standing vertically, moving, speaking, thinking
* Eating, digesting food, and other basic life functions

The body's daily energy requirements vary according to a person's age, sex and individual needs.

The Calorie Theory explains that if a particular individual needs 2,500 calories a day and consumes only 2,000, it leads to a 500 calorie deficit. To compensate for that deficit, the body will 'consume' 500 calories from existing fat reserves, which will result in losing weight.

On the other hand, if the daily intake is 3,500 calories instead of the needed 2,500, the extra 1,000 calories will automatically be stored as a body fat.

While the theory makes sense, it is too simplistic. In fact, it is purely mathematical, taken directly from Lavoisier's theory on the laws of thermodynamics. It does not take into consideration that each human body is going through its own very complex processes. Those processes depend on the age and gender, generics, hormonal, digestive and metabolic features which influence the calorie burning (or not burning) process. Also, it doesn't account for where the calories come from. According to the theory, 500 calories from cake are the same as 500 calories from cucumbers. You don't need to have a doctorate in nutrition to understand the absurdity of that statement. Everyone knows that consuming even 5,000 calories from cucumbers will never lead to gaining weight.

There are other questions as well:

* How come some people with big appetites, who consume 4,000 to 5,000 calories a day and do not have any physical activity, still stay skinny until they are elderly?

* Why do some people continue gaining weight, even when they reduce their daily calorie intake by eating much less?

Do you know such people? I do. The more overweight a person is, the more desperately he or she counts calories. They literally weigh each tiny portion, live semi-hungry and depressed, and are still not losing a pound.

On the other hand, I bet you know someone who eats EV-ERYTHING in VAST quantities and still stays very thin. I know one very elegant lady whose eating habits make me speechless. She eats huge bagels (I mean HUGE, I don't even know where she purchases them), ice cream and cakes, pota-toes, raviolis, rice — all in huge portions! It would be enough for three lunches, for me! At age 50, she is a size 2. Con-sidering the amount of calories she consumes, she should be size 20!

So, what's the catch?

The History of Calorie Theory

In 1930, two American doctors, Newburgh and Johnson, of the University of Michigan, suggested in their study that "Obesity results from a diet too high in calories, rather than from any metabolic deficiency." This was immediately and widely announced as a scientific truth, and it has been treated as a "gospel" since then.

However, the study on energy balance was based on very lim-ited data, and was conducted over too short a period of time. Continuing their study, Drs. Newburgh and Johnson came to a different conclusion a few years later, and published their con-cerns about the previous findings. The later study went entirely unnoticed. Their initial theory was already included into the pro-gram of most Western medical schools, and still remains there.

Why has the Low-Calorie approach remained so popular for almost a century!? Why do virtually all doctors, scientists and nutritionists believe in Calorie Theory and continue practicing that?

There are two explanations:

1. People DO lose weight being on a Low-Calorie diet. This is obvious. Every living creature in the world will lose weight while starving. Lack of food causes weight loss. Period. However, the fact that those results do not last very long is usually ignored. People want quick results and do not think about what happens next.

2. The second explanation is the influence of the food industry. The manufacturers are very creative and aim to give us whatever we want. Since the calorie theory is still very popular, the food manufacturers do their best to produce low-calorie food and stress the low-cal statistics on the labels and packaging. Since we are obsessed with counting calories, we get what we want. Imagine what would happen if we suddenly admitted that the calorie theory wasn't accurate and counting calories wasn't an effective weight loss strategies. Then manufacturers would stop printing the calorie numbers on the labels. Then we'd have nothing to count... Cute cycle.

Now let's see how our extra weight is explained by calorie theory.

Suppose someone needs about 2,500 calories a day and consumes that amount for years. The person's weight was fine for a while, but then something happened, and the person started to gain weight. Oh...too bad...what to do? According to the calorie theory, dropping the amount of consumed calories to

2,000 (or even less), will lead the body to use the equivalent quantity of stored fat, and the person will lose the extra weight. Sounds reasonable?

In fact, the human body is much more complicated than just a stove. If the daily intake of calories is now limited to 2,000 (instead of the 2,500 consumed for years), the body's survival instinct comes into play. It quickly adjusts its energy requirements to match the level of calorie intake: if it is only given 2,000 calories, it will only use up to 2,000 calories. Weight loss will quickly stop. The body also has an instinct for survival which will lead it to take greater precautions, and "save for a rainy day." Therefore, if it supplied with 2,000 calories, it will simply reduce its energy needs to, let's say only 1,700 calories, and store the other 300 in the form of body fat. This is exactly how we end up with achieving the very opposite result from what we want. Paradoxically, although we eat less, we gradually gain more and more weight again. After dieting, our weight not only goes back to its starting point, but in most cases we gain even more weight.

Now, stay with me. Let's say the dieting person came to the party. What are the usual thoughts?

* I've already lost 10 pounds
* I am doing well (better than John)
* It's fine to reward myself
* I deserve a prize
* That cake looks SO yummy
* Nothing is wrong if I eat a little bit more today
* I'd better skip lunch tomorrow

What's even worse is that many official diets actually RECOMMEND treating yourself! Here's where the real problems occur. In practice, the human body is constantly driven by its survival mechanisms. Compare this to the starving dog, which buries its bone. When the dog is not fed regularly, it reverts to its inborn instincts and buries its food. Staying hungry, it saves the bone for the future.

So, when our hero who already lost 10 pounds had a feast at the party, he will quickly gain weight again. His body is still "hungry" and willing to save every portion of unexpectedly received energy.

This called the Weight Cycling, also known as the yo-yo dieting effect. This name was given to that process by Kelly D. Brownell, PhD., at Yale University, in reference to the cyclical up-down motions of a yo-yo.

The story is the same. The dieter is excited about a new diet and proud of achieving quick results. Over time, the limitations cause opposite effects, such as depression or fatigue, that make the diet impossible to sustain. Also, a dieter cannot stand social events and "temporarily" gives up the diet. In addition, such emotional effects as failing to lose weight (again!), guilt and depression, lead many people to eating even more than before. They regain weight very quickly, and go back to the beginning of the cycle.

Unfortunately, this probably sounds familiar to you.

The calorie theory simply focuses on the energy value of food without paying attention to a nutritional value or particular functions of human body. However, we should admit that it is deeply embedded in our subconscious mind, and contributes into our Eating Blueprint. It is what it is, and this is where we are now.

My hope is that since you are reading this book, you are willing to UNLEARN and RELEARN, and to replace the existed blueprint with a new, healthy one. I am not saying this is easy. It won't be. It requires your desire, and commitment. You may feel confused initially, because what I am suggesting will seem odd or counterintuitive. Don't worry, you are not alone, and together we'll manage the challenge. You have a great and important goal to achieve — to reduce extra pounds if you have them, to keep your weight if you don't, to maintain a healthy lifestyle and improve your life!

Declarations:

- *I deserve to be healthy and happy*

- *I have the power to change my Eating Blueprint*

- *Nothing can hold me back on my way to success*

Chapter 2 : Roots and Fruits

"Human beings, by changing the inner attitudes
of their minds,
can change the outer aspects of their lives."
William James

*D*o you know the most common phrase I hear from people regarding their weight? "Diets don't work." I always wonder, "Haven't you reduced any pounds during three months of dieting?" "Oh, I lost 20 pounds! But they are back now."

There you go. Yo-yo dieting doesn't bring stable results, and may be even more dangerous for your health than your extra pounds. Being on a diet, you've just followed a plan. You were excited; you ate only the recommended food, exercised enthusiastically and were very happy looking at the scale. However, you did not change your attitude, your thoughts and your Eating Blueprint. You might have changed only temporarily, and that's why you got only temporary results. Be honest. Haven't you thought about eating a decent piece of cheesecake (or two-pound portion of Alfredo pasta / Donuts / Pizza / French fries) when you'll finally lose your 20 pounds? Ha! When I was on a diet, I did. I was DREAMING about that! So I did what all people do. As a reward for being strong and suffering, I ate my favorite food after dieting and…gained my favorite pounds back. I was not thinking about the roots and hidden reasons; I was worried only about results.

Understanding the relationship between reasons and results, between our inner world and outer world is beneficial. This applies to every area of our life, and is critical for success.

Our Mental World is our thoughts, emotions, beliefs, habits and spirituality influencing our Physical World. They influence our body and our behavior.

The physical realm is basically the "printout" of our inner world. The problem cannot be solved in a "printout," in our physical world. When we've already printed the paper with typo, it's too late to correct it. Again, some actions can save the situation, but it will be only a TEMPORARY solution. The error must be corrected on the computer, in a program, in our subconscious mind, thoughts, habits and beliefs. They are the roots of our outcomes.

If we aren't getting what we want in our outer life, it means that things are not going well in our inner life. Our life is a RESULT. Health is a result. Weight is a result.

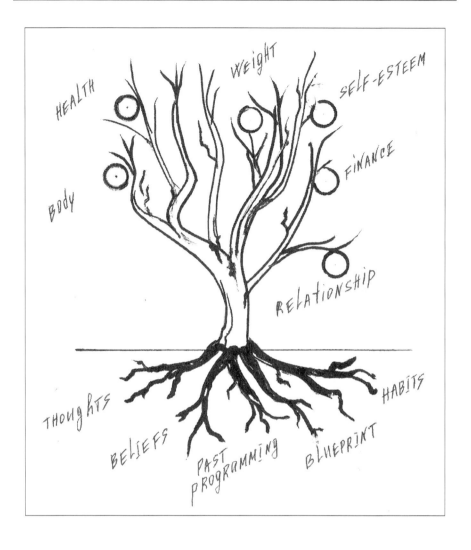

In our life, the fruits are our RESULTS. When the fruits are already on the tree, we cannot change them. However, we can analyze the roots, take actions, and change tomorrow's fruits. To harvest great fruits, we need to invest in our roots. When we treat ourselves well and have strong healthy roots, we'll get good healthy fruits. However, if we are not satisfied with our results and want to improve our life, we should change our roots to get better fruits! Think about this. It works.

Let's apply that theory to our goal of getting rid of extra pounds, being strong and healthy. What should we do? Where are those roots and how can we dig them?

The Roots of Being Overweight:

➤ Family habits
* Eating out rather than cooking at home
* Unscheduled, spontaneous meals
* Eating late at night
* Watching TV with food
* Watching TV with a drink
* Eating quick "on the fly"
* Frequently heard phrases
    ▪ "clean your plate"
    ▪ "eat to grow tall"
    ▪ "always have snacks in your bag"

➤ Food manipulations
* Food as a reward
    ▪ If you clean your room, I'll buy you an ice cream
    ▪ If you pass your test, we'll go to the Cheesecake Factory
* Food as comfort
    ▪ It's cold and rainy outside, have these fresh cookies
    ▪ Creamy soup is so cozy when it is snowing
* Food as a guilt
    ▪ Finish your food, I've spent money on that

- You are lucky to have food, many kids are starving
* Food as punishment
    - If you don't eat your breakfast, we are not going to the swimming pool
    - If you don't eat meat, dad will not buy you a bicycle

➤ Traditions

* Celebrating with a lot of food
* Entertaining with a lot of food

➤ Media

* Buying advertised food
* Eating in advertised restaurants
* Following celebrities' diets

➤ Society

* Buying discounted food
* Using all possible coupons
* Buying big packages to save money
* Eating for free at work
* Eating much more in a buffet

➤ Anger, nervous

* Eating frequently
* Eating more
* Eating snacks and junk food
* Eating food that usually not eaten in other situations
* Drinking more soft and alcoholic beverages

➣ Just for spite
  * Eating even more enthusiastically when people are looking at your huge portion
  * Eating more when someone advises you to diet

➣ Low self-esteem
  * I am not worthy anyway
  * This is the only joy I have
  * When I eat I feel better

➣ Playing a victim
  * I have bad genes
  * I was born like this
  * I will never be like her/him anyway
  * I just have low metabolism
  * My life is so hard

➣ Ignorance
  * I don't care
  * I'll eat what I want, don't tell me what to eat
  * Life is short
  * I am still OK
  * I am slimmer than her/him
  * Food can't cause a disease

➣ Inaccurate Beliefs
  * Counting calories and focusing on food quantity rather than quality
  * Fat people are more kind and happy
  * Fat people have more energy
  * Fat people are healthier
  * Healthy food is expensive

* I need carbs for energy
* I need my sugar portion, it is good for my muscles
* I need my coffee to keep me up

➢ Lack of nutrition knowledge
  * Not understanding the basic principles of fat metabolism
  * Not understanding food categories
  * Not understanding food combinations
  * Not paying attention to ingredients on the food labels

I remember how my grandma was standing at the door and saying, "You are not going to school until you finish your breakfast!" I don't know if it was a punishment or a reward, but I went back to the table and finished (or at least had some more) breakfast. Believe it or not, breakfast is still the most important meal for me. I never leave my home without eating breakfast. I LOVE having breakfast at restaurants, or cooking fancy breakfasts for my friends and family.

So, what do you think? Do you recognize this pattern in your life? Did you find any single root there? A few? Congratulations! The more you found, the more chances for success you have! Are they healthy roots or harmful roots? You are already on your way to treating the unhealthy roots, to straightening the healthy ones, and then to grow fabulous fruits to enjoy them forever!

Food Categories

As we already know, we gain weight not because we eat a lot, but because we have bad eating habits. It's not about quantity; it's about the quality of the food. I will be the last person to tell you DO NOT eat. I enjoy parties, family gatherings, cozy and comfort eating, fancy restaurants and elegant romantic dinners. Food is a huge part of our life. It brings joy, fixes the mood and contributes to relationships. Our purpose is not to DECLINE food, but to CHOOSE the right ones. Make a right choice for every occasion.

So, how can we choose the food that we need? It starts from understanding the food categories. When we know which particular category to choose from, we can make the right choices and maintain a desired healthy lifestyle.

Let me take you on a little tour about the origins of food, and present it to you in a simple and easy way, so you'll remember it.

All food products contain certain amount of basic subsets as fats, proteins and carbohydrates. Also, in each product there are minerals and vitamins, water and cellulose fiber.

Proteins are the organic base of every life material. All our organs, muscles and bones are built from proteins. Proteins are also built from more simple chemical elements, called monoacids. Some of them are produced by our body, and some we get from food. Proteins within food may be animal or plant based.

Animal based proteins:
* Meat
* Fish
* Cheese
* Eggs
* Milk products

Plant based proteins:
* Soya
* Nuts
* Some grains
* Beans

Proteins are very important materials for:
* Building cells and as a potential source of energy after transformation to glucose.
* Producing some hormones
* Producing nuclear acids which are necessary for reproduction.

Deficit of proteins may lead to such illnesses as muscle weakness, immune deficiencies, wrinkling of the skin and skin diseases. Excluding eggs, non-animal or plant proteins do not support the necessary balance of amino acids in the body. Deficit of one amino acid may lead to difficulties in absorption of others. That is why your food should contain proteins from both animals and plants. Vegetarian food with only plant proteins is not balanced and may lead to nail and hair problems. However, a vegetarian diet which includes eggs and milk products is healthy and supports the necessary food balance.

Carbohydrates are those substances which molecules are built from molecules of carbon, oxygen and hydrogen. During the chemical process, they convert to glucose. Carbohydrates can be classified by their molecular structure:

* *Mono-carbohydrates* — carbohydrates which have only one molecule
    * Glucose (included in honey and fruits)
    * Fructose (included in honey and fruits)
    * Gluten (included in milk)

* *Double carbohydrates* — carbohydrates which have two molecules
    * Sucrose from white sugar or beets and cane sugar
    * Lactose from milk
    * Maltose from beer and corn

* Carbohydrates from several molecules
    * Glycogen in animal's liver
    * Starch, included in such food as wheat, corn, rice, potatoes, beets, beans and soy.

All carbohydrates can be characterized as "bad" and "good" based on their ability to influence blood sugar. I will explain this impact in the next chapter.

Lipids are also known as fat acids. Depending on their origin, they may be divided into animal or plant based.

Lipids from animal tissue:
* Meat
* Fish

* Butter
* Eggs
* Cheese
* Cream

Lipids from plants:

* Peanut
* Olive
* Walnut
* Margarine

Also, because their molecules are more complex, lipids may be classified by their chemical structure. There are three big lipid categories:

Saturated lipids, from:

* Meat
* Kielbasa
* Whole milk
* Butter
* Cream
* Cheese

Monounsaturated lipids, from:

* Olive oil
* Goose and duck oil
* Goose liver

Polyunsaturated lipids, oils from:

* Nuts, fruits and vegetables
* Fish and shellfish

Fats are very important for the human body. They create reserves of energy which our body uses when necessary; they're included in the cells of many tissues and organs, particularly in the central nervous system. Fats contain different vitamins (A, D, E, K) and fatty acids that produce different hormones.

Fats can be also categorized by their influence on the level of blood cholesterol.

Fats that are responsible for the high level of blood cholesterol and have saturated fat acids include:

* Meat
* Kielbasa
* Butter
* Cheese
* Pork fat
* Whole milk products
* Palm oil

Some fats which don't affect the level of cholesterol include:

* Shellfish
* Eggs
* Poultry with the skin removed

And some fats may even decrease the cholesterol level in the blood. These are vegetable oils:

* Olive oil
* Rapeseed oil
* Sunflower oil
* Corn oil

As for fish oils, they don't play a major role in cholesterol metabolism, but they do help prevent cardiovascular disease by decreasing the level of triglycerides and preventing blood clots. The oilier the fish, the better it is for our health:

* Salmon
* Tuna
* Mackerel
* Herrings
* Sardines

Cellulose fiber does not have any energetic potential, but plays a very important role in food digestion and normal functioning of our body. It is found in vegetables, beans, fruits and grains and enriched with vitamins, microelements and minerals. It also decreases the toxic effect of some chemicals, preservatives or food colors, and prevents some gastrointestinal tract diseases.

All four groups of food are important for balanced and healthy nutrition and should be included in certain amounts in our everyday diet. However, for our purpose of achieving and keeping a healthy weight, let's divide them into two big groups:

The categories which are NOT responsible for the pounds we gain:

* Proteins
* Cellulose fiber

The categories which are RESPONSIBLE for the pounds we gain:

* Carbohydrates
* Lipids

As you can see, the blame for "those extra pounds" is attributable to carbohydrates and fats, though not all types of them.

As a general rule, we eat too much carbohydrates and fatty food, especially deep fried food, French fries, chips, doughnuts, a wide variety of sweets and soft drinks, or unnecessary heavy sauces. Now, when we understand the food categories and can differentiate between "good" and "bad" food, we can easily choose the positive inputs over the unhealthy ones. In the subsequent chapters, I will show you how to build healthy eating habits and to replace harmful foods with beneficial ones in everyday meals. I will show you that healthy cooking is fun, and the food is just as delicious as the "unhealthy" foods you have been consuming.

How and why we gain weight

This part of the book may seem to you as the most complicated and "too scientific," but I have included this information here to explain the very basics of our fat metabolism. Many people prefer quick-results-diets or magic pills over a lifestyle nutrition. We are happy to show BEFORE and AFTER results, in spite of the fact that very soon after our AFTER results, we are back to BEFORE. Doesn't matter! We'll do that again! We are ready for a new (very popular!) quick-results-diets or (just discovered!) magic pill. We excitedly run into that and … fail again for the long term. We have more photos for the 'BE-FORE and AFTER' album.

I think that one of the main reasons for failure in maintaining a healthy lifestyle is not being aware of the functions of the human body. Don't worry; you don't need to apply to medical school to know that, unless you want to. Just read this part of the chapter patiently and reread it periodically. I strongly believe that when we clearly picture what happens inside of our body, we can influence our health. This is also the best motivation we can ever have. So, PLEASE be patient and READ the following pages.

Why and how we gain weight? What actually happens when we eat?

Whether or not we accumulate fat is directly related to the hormone insulin. This is not the ONLY mechanism, but the main one.

Insulin is produced by beta-cells of the pancreas, and plays the major role in regulating carbohydrate and fat metabolism. It stimulates uptake of glucose (sugar) from the blood to the cells in the body. The glucose may then be used for our energy needs, or stored as a body fat.

In a healthy person, insulin releases in two phases. Small portions of insulin are continually going out of the pancreas to remove glucose from the blood, regardless of the sugar level. In addition, the pancreas increases the insulin secretion when sugar level is up (after a carbohydrate meal). When there is no new sugar in the blood and its level is low, the body begins to use fat as an energy source.

When the pancreas is healthy, the amount of produced insulin is proportional to the amount of glucose in the blood to deal with. However, if the pancreas is defective, it releases greater amounts of insulin than is needed to handle the particular amount of glucose. This causes glucose to be stored as fat instead of being used for energy needs.

As you age, the body cells that remove glucose from the blood may become less sensitive (more resistant) to the insulin. This condition is called insulin resistance. An estimated 10 to 15 percent of adults in the United States have insulin resistance.

Since the body cells do not react on normally produced amounts of insulin, the pancreas starts producing much more insulin than normal. High levels of insulin in the blood is called hyperinsulinemia.

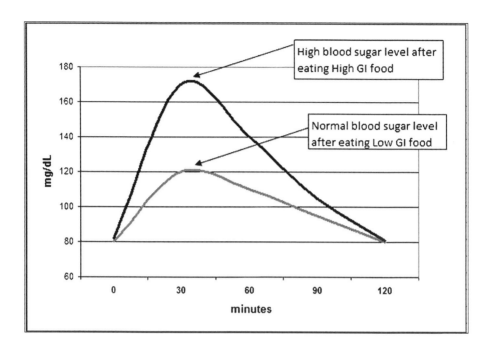

For example, if in a normal person, 1 unit of insulin might be needed to help 10 mg of glucose go into the cell, then in a hyper-insulinemic person, 10 units of insulin might be needed to get the same 10 mg of glucose into the cell. That high blood level of insulin may remain asymptomatic for many years. If so, why should we care about that? First, because the high level of insulin decreases the blood sugar level, and people may feel such symptoms as:

* Temporary muscle weakness
* Brain fog
* Fatigue
* Temporary thought disorder, or inability to concentrate
* Headaches

* Shaking/trembling
* Thirst

Second, the hyper production of insulin and insulin resistance of body cells can lead to health problems, and put us at risk of more serious conditions such as:

* High level of blood triglycerides (lipids) which increase the risk of heart attack and stroke

* High risk of blood vessels clotting

* Low HDL cholesterol (the good one, which we want to be higher) increases risk of heart attack and stroke

* High uric acid (the disease called gout, also known as podagra)

* Polycystic ovary syndrome (women's endocrine disorder with period problems, infertility, excessive beard and chest hairiness, and obesity)

* Type 2 diabetes

* Obesity

* High blood pressure

I don't mean to scare you, but if we want to be healthy, we need to know our enemies.

As we can see, it is mostly the condition of the pancreas, insulin secretion and insulin resistance that determine whether a person will gain weight or not. The person who easily gains weight simply has a tendency to hyper-insulinemia.

Declarations:

- *I make smart choices*

- *I know the difference between food categories*

- *I know how my body works*

Chapter 3 : Unlearn and Relearn

*"The illiterate of the 21st century will not be those
who cannot read and write,
but those who cannot learn, unlearn, and relearn."*

Alvin Toffler

Now, once you become aware of the weak roots of your Eating Blueprint, you are willing to grow healthy ones, right?

There is an old Chinese story about a teacher and a student. The student refused to accept a new theory, was arguing with the teacher and declining his every word. The teacher did not become angry; he simply asked the student if he would like to have some tea. Then he took a full cup of tea and put it on the table in front of the student. Immediately, he took a tea-pot and started to fill the cup which was already full. Hot tea spilled over the table and the floor. The student was stunned and yelled, "What are you doing?!! Don't you see? The cup is already full!" The teacher replied, "This is exactly what I wanted to show you. To put fresh tea in your cup, you should empty your cup first. When your cup is empty, more fresh tea can fit there."

This is about the "unlearn" principle. When we are full of our old beliefs, there is no space for new ones. It does not mean that we need to discard all our previous experience and knowledge. It just means that we need to be open to analyzing them. Obviously, it's perfect when our previous experience is helping by bringing us success and happiness. Our knowledge serves us and there is no need to get rid of it. However, what happens if we are stuck and nothing works in our favor anymore? What if we are not satisfied with today's results and want to move to a higher level of life? That's when it's time to let old beliefs go and adopt new ones. Yes, we need to be open-minded towards unlearning, learning and relearning. It's true that changes take time and nothing happens overnight. It requires lots of energy, efforts and coordinated actions on a regular basis. Sometimes, a new idea sounds so odd that you can't even consider taking it seriously. However, when you analyze the past and relearn, you may find a new way extremely effective and beneficial indeed. Therefore, having a flexible and open mindset towards unlearning and relearning is important. When you keep following your main purpose, your passion will make the process easier and you'll enjoy it. The desire to be healthy will feed your goal of achieving the ideal weight. Your healthy and energetic body will support your renewed self-esteem, and you'll discover that you have become more confident and attractive. When you're passionate about your desire, you will find that it will bring you amazing results in every area of your life: professional development, finances, family and relationships, and your emotional and spiritual life. Consider your current beliefs about yourself, your health, your body and your eating habits. Unlearn first, and then replace old beliefs with those that will take you closer to your goal!

"Live as if you were to die tomorrow. Learn as if you were to live forever."
- Mahatma Gandhi

The Glycemic Index

"A primary method for gaining a mind full of peace is to practice emptying the mind."
Napoleon Hill

Now we know "who is guilty in those extra pounds":

* Some hereditary conditions
* The existed eating habits, called Eating Blueprint
* "Bad" carbohydrates and "bad" lipids
* Hyper production of hormone insulin by pancreas

How can we apply that knowledge to our everyday life?

On this list, the only one thing that you cannot change is your genes, your hereditary conditions. The other factors can be managed, and that is very good news. By fixing them, you'll be able to decrease risk factors of many diseases, get healthier and more energetic, learn how to make better choices and enjoy eating, cooking, entertaining and socializing without putting yourself and your loved ones in risk. There is only one person who can do that – YOU. Let's move forward and learn more about carbohydrates and how to differentiate the 'good' carbs from the 'bad' ones.

I want to introduce you to the Low Glycemic Index nutrition principles which can help you make your choices easier every day.

The Glycemic Index Definition.

According to the School of Molecular and Microbial Biosciences at the University of Sydney, the Glycemic Index (GI) is "a ranking of carbohydrates on a scale from 0 to 100 according to the extent to which they raise blood sugar levels after eating." In other words, it is the potential of each carbohydrate to increase blood sugar levels. The GI was initially formulated by Dr. David Jenkins at the University of Toronto and first used in 1976 in creating a special diet for diabetic patients. Nowadays, many institutions around the World continue to investigate the GI of food and its influence on human health.

The Sydney University GI Research Service was established in 1995 and provides laboratory testing for the local and international food industry. The GI of food is tested on a group of 8 to 12 healthy volunteers. They consume food with a fixed portion of carbohydrates, usually 50 grams. The actual portion size of each tested food varies, because different foods contain different amount of carbohydrates. For example, if carrots contain only about 7% of carbs, the portion of carrots will be about 1.5 pounds. However, the cooked spaghetti contains 25% carbohydrates; therefore, to supply 50 gram of carbohydrates with spaghetti, the volunteer is given a portion of about a half of pound. Then, the blood tests are taken every 15-30 minutes, and a two hour trend graph is created for the sugar level.

To reflect the total increase in blood sugar after eating the test food, the area under the curve is calculated. The glucose is used as the reference food, and the GI of other carbohydrates is calculated using the following formula:

$$\frac{\text{Area below curve for the carbohydrate tested}}{\text{Area below curve for glucose}} \times 100$$

The average response from volunteers will determine the GI of tested food. The higher the blood sugar average after consuming the particular carbohydrate, the higher will be its Glycemic Index.

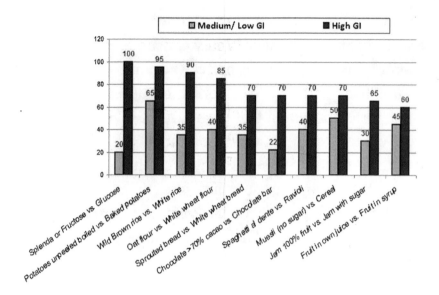

The GI measurement applies only to food that contains carbohydrates. Since lipids and proteins do not contain carbohydrates, they do not have a GI. The glucose is used as a specific benchmark and given a GI of 100 by definition. The GI greater than 50 is considered as High GI, 35-50 is a Medium GI, lower than 35 is a Low GI. The GI Table found at the end of the book will provide you with more detailed information about the GI of different types of food.

Various factors influence the GI of food:

* Chemical processing
* Cooking methods
* Ripeness of food
* Amount of the cellulose fiber
* Quality of the cellulose fiber
* Food temperature
* Food variety

For example, fried potatoes have a GI of 95, while the GI of potatoes boiled with the skin is 70. White bread has a GI of 90, and multigrain bread has a GI of 50. White rice is 70, and wild rice is 50.

Today, low GI nutrition is widely practiced in Europe, Australia and New Zealand. In the US, several diet plans such as Atkins, South Beach and Warrior are based on GI principles.

Personally, I find the GI approach easy to follow, and not any harder than other diets. It has both advantages and disadvantages. What do you want first: good news or bad news? Let's start from the negatives:

Disadvantages of the Low GI nutrition:

* May be difficult for people who feel they are addicted to carbohydrates

* May be difficult for athletes, because they need a much larger energy input than non-athletes

* Does not bring quick results

* Should be considered as a long-term lifestyle, not a temporary diet

Advantages of the Low GI nutrition:

* Focuses on maintaining healthy functioning of pancreas

* Lowers blood levels of sugar, insulin, cholesterol and triglycerides

* Prevents many life-threatening diseases

* The results are stable and last for years

* Is nutritionally balanced

* Requires no calorie counting

* Requires no portions control

* Is based on consuming healthy (not saturated) fat and healthy carbohydrates

* Is suitable for vegetarians who eat eggs and milk products

* Provides food replacement strategies for favorite recipes

* Allows periodic food rewards on special occasions (if you still want them)

My purpose is to explain how to use a basic approach following low GI nutrition, because it will help you maintain a healthy weight without following a specific diet. When you can easily choose between different food categories and different GI foods, you will be able to maintain YOUR OWN healthy nutrition style and follow it for years. You won't have to follow some other diet program any longer.

I'll now examine carbohydrates in more detail. This food category requires special attention, because weight gain comes primarily from eating the wrong carbohydrates, or eating them in combination with certain foods.

To make it simple, divide all carbohydrates into two big groups:

* Carbohydrates with a low GI, or GOOD carbohydrates
* Carbohydrates with a high GI, or BAD carbohydrates

Bad carbohydrates are those that have high GI, lead to a significant increase in blood sugar and, as a result, to a significant insulin secretion. Basically, each of them can be assigned to one of the following:

* Sugar
* White flour
* Starch

These are "three elephants" responsible for weight gain. I think that sugar should be labeled with a skull-and-crossbones symbol, like other lethal substances. Some 200 years ago sugar was still a luxury and not available to most people. For millions of years, people lived without it and they were healthy, productive and created great scientific and cultural masterpieces. In addition to adding extra pounds, sugar is a major cause of diabetes, chronic fatigue, gastrointestinal issues, cavities and heart diseases. This applies to pure sugar in any form, and to all products which include it: such as soda, cookies, cakes, etc.

All products which include white flour and starch are also considered 'bad' carbohydrates and cause weight gain and diseases.

Unlike "bad" carbohydrates, the "good" carbohydrates are those which are only partially absorbed by the body, lead to much smaller elevation in blood sugar levels, and as a result, to smaller insulin secretion. This group includes whole grains, beans, most fruits, and all vegetables.

Your goal should be to learn to switch "bad" carbs with "good" carbs, or with foods that are high in proteins and healthy fats. It is about quality versus quantity.

Changing your Eating Blueprint requires knowledge, patience and time. Don't simply say you refuse to make changes. Take your time and THINK about it. When you come to the right conclusions by yourself, the transformation will be easier and you'll do it with much less effort.

It took me about two months to digest the theory, change my Eating Blueprint and start to apply the low GI nutrition principles to my everyday life. Since then, I have successfully followed it for 15 years and I will never give it up. I have maintained my ideal weight and have kept it very easily; I eat gourmet food and enjoy social events, love cooking and entertaining friends.

Are you willing to stop dieting, become healthier and improve your life?

Eating Habits that kill the pancreas

The healthy pancreas is the main factor that distinguishes overweight healthy people, or people who don't eat much and still gain weight, from people who eat "whatever they see" and still stay slim.

In many cases this condition is hereditary, but it can still be managed by proper diet. Also, preventing the risk of diseases in hereditary conditions becomes even more important. Let's analyze eating habits that begin in early childhood.

As young children, we like to drink sweet sodas, eat cookies, candies, marshmallows, ice cream, pancakes, muffins, macaroni & cheese, pizza and French fries. We eat these foods on a daily basis or as an occasional treat or reward, depending on the family rules and Eating Blueprint. Have you ever offered a celery stick, instead of an ice cream cone, to a crying child? I've never seen that and don't think I ever will.

At school, children carry cookies or chocolate bars for snacks, then have mashed potatoes, pizza, pasta or rice at home, and drink soda during the entire day.

At college, we eat sandwiches and hamburgers from the fast food place around the corner, pizza and French fries again. Weekends are full of a lot of beer and "all you can eat" Chinese buffets with foods full of sugar and starch.

Once we start working and earning some money, the quality of our meals may improve, but we are still the prisoners of our Eating Blueprint. Sandwiches are still very popular and quick. Also, many offices have pantries or coffee areas featuring free donuts and muffins which look (and maybe even taste) SO good.

If we are going out for dinner, we prefer skipping lunch "to decrease calorie intake." We feel weak, hungry and angry; we think that we need our caffeine portion and drink one cup of a strong coffee after another, usually with sugar.

Weekends bring pub meals with friends or traditional family gatherings with barbecues, baked potatoes, sweet corn, and (of course!) plenty of beer and sweet soda.

That is the story of how we almost kill our pancreas by the age of 35 to 40. And, this is exactly the age when we find ourselves "suddenly" overweight.

It is also the story of how we become addicted to the unhealthy foods and to the bad carbohydrates. They stimulate the pancreas to produce more and more insulin and the body stores more and more fat.

Hopefully, you're still reading and focused on how to make changes in your diet. After such a brain-washing, you might throw this book away and order a double cheese pizza. If you haven't done so, you are a winner, and "winners never quit." It's time to invest in your well-being by getting rid of those unhealthy addictions and extra pounds.

The aforementioned is a general description of a **Bad Eating Cycle**, and here is a full picture:

* We eat bad carbs (cookie, donut, muffin, waffle with maple syrup, etc.). It's delicious; we've got our sugar portion, we are full and happy.

* However, our body doesn't think so...The blood sugar level is too high now, and beats the pancreas

* The pancreas is not happy either, and sends its angry response by producing a huge amount of insulin

* Insulin is always ready to help and enthusiastically reduces the blood sugar level

* The blood sugar cannot stand the charming insulin and drops dramatically without even fighting

* However, our body is not happy again...We experience weakness, fatigue, hunger and even brain fog. We are upset and in a bad mood. We must work to be productive; we want our profits; we desperately need our sugar level up! So we have another cup of very strong coffee (with sugar of course!) and just a tiny-mini (or not) cookie (muffin, donut or brownie).

* We ate that, it was delicious, we've got our sugar back, we fixed our mood and perhaps even our potential profits, we are full and happy.

* However, out body doesn't think so AGAIN...The blood sugar level is too high now, and beats the pancreas

* The pancreas is not happy either, and sends its angry response by producing a huge amount of insulin

The cycle goes on and on....

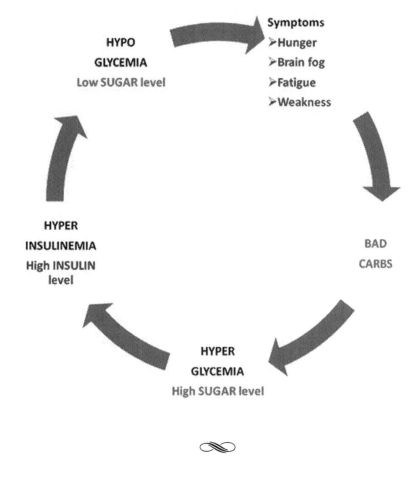

Declarations:

- *I am getting rid of my wrong beliefs*

- *My bad nutrition habits are in the past*

- *I am committed to constantly learning and growing*

Cnnno

The Recipe of the Chapter:

Juicy Portobello Mushrooms

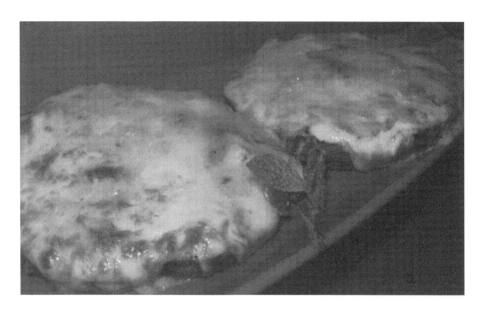

Mushrooms contain fiber and have a low Glycemic Index of only 15. They can be combined with proteins and lipids (cheese, mayonnaise) or other vegetables (tomatoes). They're perfect for a light but nourishing dinner, or romantic evening. Feel free to add fresh salad and variety of cheese. Red or white wine will highlight the taste.

4 Portobello mushrooms. They should be not too large or too thick. This way they cook particularly tender and juicy.

For stuffing:
2 tomatoes
1/3 pound of horseradish cheese
Mayonnaise (no sugar no starch added)
Salt, pepper and thyme (if desired).

Clean mushrooms with a dry paper towel. Take off the stems and arrange mushrooms on the baking sheet or into a baking dish. Sprinkle them with salt and pepper.

Cut tomatoes into thin slices and simmer in frying pan on low heat for 4 to 5 minutes. Add some salt and pepper. In each mushroom cup put one teaspoon of mayonnaise, add in the cooked tomatoes and grated cheese. You may add some thyme and/or fresh ground pepper on top.

Bake 15 minutes in a toaster oven, or regular oven at 450*F.

If you bake them in a fancy baking dish, serve them right away. If you bake them on a baking sheet, move them carefully with a wide spatula to a serving dish.

Chapter 4 : Past programming

"Consciousness is observing your thoughts and actions so that you can live from true choice in the present moment rather than being run by programming from the past."
T. Harv Eker

Let me share with you an extremely powerful formula taught by many respected Personal Development gurus. I first heard about this at T. Harv Eker Peak Potentials Training, and was impressed with how wise it is. The formula is called "The Process of Manifestation" and is presented this way:

Thoughts→Feelings→Actions→Results

➢ **T**houghts lead to Feelings
➢ **F**eelings lead to Actions
➢ **A**ctions lead to **R**esults

The next question is – where do our thoughts come from? Why does each of us think differently? Why are her thoughts different from his thoughts and his thoughts are not the same as mine?

It brings us back to the Blueprint point. Early in your life and during your childhood, many different ideas were installed in your mind from outside sources. Those ideas were absorbed and stored. This process can be compared to creating and saving computer files. First, the programmer created a code, ran it, exported files and saved them in a certain folder. Then those files were used by a person. Is our behavior any different? Not really. We think and act according to the previously installed files, to the initial 'programming.' Our past programming determines our current thoughts and actions.

If we add that programming part to the Process of Manifestation formula, we will get:

Past Programming→Thoughts→Feelings→Actions→Results

> ➣ **P**rogramming leads to **T**houghts
>> ➣ **T**houghts lead to **F**eelings
>> ➣ **F**eelings lead to **A**ctions
>> ➣ **A**ctions lead to **R**esults

When we replace files and make program changes in our personal computer, we receive a different outcome. The same is true about us. As a first step toward changing our results, we need to change the programming and replace the old files in our mind with new or updated ones.

Now, how does that programming happen? It comes from each of our five senses: what we hear, see, smell, touch or taste, and from our own specific experience.

What was YOUR experience when you were young?

* What did you hear about food when you were young?
* What did you see when you were young?
* What did you experience when you were young?
* What were your family eating habits?
* Did food mean entertainment?
* Did entertainment mean food?
* What kind of food was popular in your home?
* What kind of breakfast? Lunch? Dinner?
* Did family members eat together?
* Were you accustomed to 'speed eating on the fly' or did you savor your meals?
* Did you eat mostly fast food or homemade food?
* How were family events related to food?
* What did you hear about diets?
* Were family members following any diets?
* What were the results?

How do you eat now?

* Do you eat because you are hungry, or because you SEE the food around?

* Do you eat until you are full, or until you finish all food available?

* Do you eat while entertaining friends, or because you feel lonely?

Thinking about this topic and answering those questions may uncover hidden roots of unhealthy (or healthy) eating habits.

One of my clients (we'll call her Ms. A) provided me with a good example of stress release programming.

Ms. A. is a beautiful 35 year old woman who wants to be healthy and improve her shape. She is not overweight, is interested in healthy nutrition, and does her best to choose the appropriate foods. However, she has a destructive habit of eating junk food (and a lot of it!) when she's under stress. When we discussed her childhood and her family, we quickly uncovered the root for this behavior. She is the youngest child in a family, and she has two older brothers. She was loved by all family members and grew up laughing and happy. However, like all children, there were times when this lovely little girl got upset or was crying. What did her parents (and grandparents of course) do every time when she was crying? They ran to her with a food treat (do you remember 'Food as a Treat' root?). "Oh, poor baby, let's get you an ice cream!" (Think chips, pizza, hamburger, cheesecake, muffin and so on). By the way, it's pretty hard to imagine using an apple, or baby-carrots for such a treat.

OK, the baby grows up and becomes a beautiful smart woman. Again, every time something upsets her, she treats herself with guess what? Right! With an ice cream, chips, pizza, hamburger, cheesecake, muffin, etc! She got that idea from her parents and grandparents; she saw how it was practiced in her family, and she experienced it. The blueprint is so strong that even after 30 years she continues to practice the same behavior. The good news is that now she is AWARE and wants to change her past programming. We'll talk more about that in the upcoming chapters, but now let's look at the exact opposite example of programmed behavior.

Once, when Ms. B was three years old, she had a difficulty breathing while eating raspberries. It lasted for just several minutes, but seriously scared her and her parents. They took their daughter to the doctors who ran some tests; however, the real cause of that short breathing still wasn't clear. As a precaution, her mother started to check carefully the ingredients of juices, ice cream and other food to see whether they contained raspberries. Since then, Ms. B never experienced the shortening of breath, but the file "raspberries are bad for me" was strongly embedded in her mind. Do you think she ever touched raspberries again? NEVER in her entire life. Not raspberries or raspberry juice, chocolate with raspberries, raspberry cake, jelly or ice cream. NEVER.

Now, wouldn't it be great to install "candies are bad for me" (cookies, donuts, cakes, chips, popcorn or fried food) files deeply in our subconscious? Don't you think it would be incredibly helpful? If only!

Some programming can be even more harmful. Imagine a child who watches his dad drinking beer throughout the evening as he watches TV. If the show is 30 minutes, he drinks just one beer. When he watches several hours of TV, he drinks…you name it. What are the chances that the child will do the same when he grows up? Obviously very high. In this case, it is not just about a bad habit, but also about addiction to alcohol, which no one would wish on anyone. We may think that a toddler doesn't pay attention and doesn't understand what we eat and drink, but it is just not true. The files for modeling parents' behavior are easily installed at a very young age and spread deep roots very quickly. Those roots will produce unhealthy fruits, and then we need to dig deeper and harder to treat them in order to grow different, nice and healthy fruits.

Research has shown that young babies know naturally when they are hungry and when they've already had enough to eat. They just stop eating as soon as they are full. However, later on that begins to change. We develop habits which cause us to eat even when we basically don't need food and aren't hungry. We eat too much because we are happy or unhappy, alone or have company, reading or watching TV, or even because we find the packaging of a particular meal or snack appealing. Sounds familiar, doesn't it?

Eating while watching TV is a very popular "bad eating habit," In fact, it is not about the "eating while watching TV" habit, but about "eating WHAT while watching TV" habit.

I'd be the last person to advise you NOT to eat in front of the TV or other family gatherings. Family evenings are important and no one wants to miss those precious moments of togetherness. But, we can fully enjoy these moments using the replacement strategies for food servings.

Why do you think that popcorn, potato chips, pizza and beer are the best options for family evenings? It's simple—you are used to this food. Because you saw, heard and experienced that starting in your childhood, because this is the way it was in your family, your friends' families, at school and college, and this is what you absorbed from media and commercials. But you want to be healthy, be a good example to your kids or grandkids. You definitely want THEM to be healthy, and the best – you are still reading this book. So, let's think together how can we enjoy our warm family evenings and achieve our healthy goals. Next time when your family sits together, try to arrange the following items on the table:

* All kinds of berries and fruits such as fresh strawberries and pineapple

* All kinds of nuts (not roasted in honey or sugar, please)

* Baby carrots, cut sweet peppers in all colors and other vegetables of your choice

* Assorted types of cheese

* Chocolate with more than 70% cacao. The GI of such chocolate is only 20 and does not lead to gaining weight

* Fresh squeezed fruit or vegetable juices

* Dry red wine for adults if desired

I'm sure that you would agree these are all appealing substitutes for popcorn, chips and beer.

To conclude this chapter about the power of our past programming, I would like to tell you the story about Grandma's Cooking Family Secret.

The new bride makes her first dinner for her husband's family according to her mother's recipe. She carefully places potato slices, carrots and onions around the dish. Then she takes a big piece of ham, cuts off the edges and puts the rest in the pan. Her husband thinks that meat is delicious and asks, "Why did you throw away good pieces of meat?" She replied. "That's the way my mother always did it."

Next time, the young couple went to her parents for dinner and the husband was watching how his mother-in-law was cooking. She carefully placed potato slices, carrots and onions. Then she took a big piece of ham, cut off the edges and put the rest in the pan. "May I ask you why you threw away good pieces of meat?" asked the young son-in-law gently. She replied, "That's the way my mother always did it."

Next time, when the couple went to the grandmother for dinner, the young husband decided to uncover that family secret and was watching closely how she was making the dinner. She placed potato slices, carrots and onions in the pan. Then she took a big piece of ham, put it in the pan as well, and then placed everything in the oven. Holding his breath, he asked, "Grandma, didn't you forget something?" "What darling?

What could I forget? I have cooked it like this for decades. No, everything is fine." "Are you sure? Don't you need to cut the ham's edges?" Grandma was confused and quiet for a minute, then she laughed and replied, "Oh, that! No, my darling, I now have a bigger pan!"

Declarations:

- *I am ready to get rid of my unhealthy eating habits*

- *I am happily building my new healthy lifestyle*

- *I love my body and feed it with healthy and delicious food*

ᏬᏬᏬ

The Recipe of the Chapter:

Colorful and Flavorful Ham and Cheese Appetizers

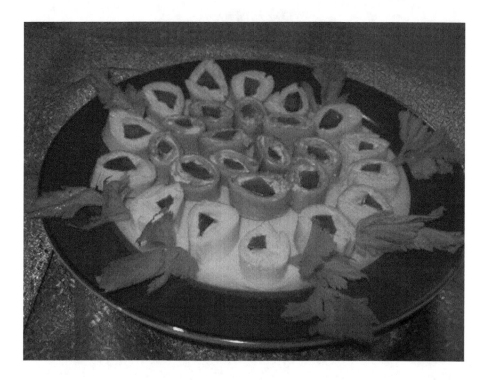

This appetizer does not contain bad carbohydrates. It is a combination of proteins, lipids and fiber. The GI of pickles and red peppers is only 15 and they go well with both cheese and meat. The dish looks smells and tastes great!

Ingredients:
6 slices of ham (about 4x4 inches)
6 slices of horseradish cheese (about 4x4 inches)
1 package (8oz) of low fat cream cheese
1-2 pickles (or marinated cucumbers) cut into thin long strips
1 red pepper cut into thin long strips

For ham appetizers:
Spread cream cheese over each slice of ham, put one strip of pickle on the edge and roll up tightly, pressing to seal.

For cheese appetizers:
Spread cream cheese over each slice of cheese, put one strip of red pepper on the edge and roll up tightly, pressing to seal.

Put ham and cheese rolls in separate containers and let them stay in the refrigerator for 8-16 hours.

Before serving, cut each roll into 5-6 pieces (about ½ inch each) and place them all together on a serving dish.

Chapter 5 : Count Thoughts not Calories

"Watch your thoughts; they become words.
Watch your words; they become actions.
Watch your actions; they become habits.
Watch your habits; they become character.
Watch your character; it becomes your destiny"
Frank Outlaw

People pay less attention to being overweight than to obesity, probably because of the aesthetic view, not from the perspective of health. In fact, people KNOW they eat too much of the wrong foods, but prefer to ignore that fact and do nothing about it. Many of us accept yo-yo dieting almost as a lifestyle, in spite of gaining even more pounds after each attempt.

According to statistics, 66% of adults in the US are overweight or obese. Every year, obesity causes about 112,000 deaths from cardiovascular disease, more than 15,000 deaths related to cancer, and more than 35,000 deaths to other diseases. It is scary and sad, because the majority of those deaths could be prevented.

When people make a decision "to be on a diet," they do it mostly because of social or personal events, such as meeting a new boyfriend or girlfriend, attending their own or someone else's wedding, summer season (to fit into a bikini), birthday, holiday season, looking for a new job, etc. So, as we can see, they are mostly "I don't like myself as I am now" reasons. The reason "I want to be healthy" is much rarer, and mostly appears when something negative has already happened. Such as a diagnosis of high blood sugar or/and cholesterol, pancreas or liver disease, abnormal ECG or positive stress test, etc. Why should we wait for these dangerous signs? Why is being able to fit into a dress or suit and look 10 pounds thinner more important than being healthy and living longer?

The bottom line of "I need to fit into the dress (suit)" is "I am fat and ugly now. If I am slimmer – I'll be more attractive." This is an extremely negative starting point. According to the Law of Attraction, we attract more negative things into our life by thinking negatively. Even if we lose those extra pounds by that wedding, we'll gain more of them very soon and be back to the initial point "I am fat and ugly now, I need to be slimmer to be more attractive." Is this what you want? Do you want to be back to your BEFORE, when you have already achieved your AFTER?

However, such thoughts as "I desire to be healthy, beautiful, attractive and energetic" or "I want to live a long healthy life and be a great example to my loved ones" sound different. They give you the powerful motivating and positive approach that includes envisioning a future with your healthy body, soul, relationships and your whole life. I think this image is worth having and you should know that you deserve it.

The Power of Positive Thinking

Positive thinking means talking and thinking about what you DESIRE, and not about something that you DON'T want. Listen to people around you. They talk endlessly about their problems and probably enjoy doing so. They hardly discuss anything inspiring and motivational, or share stories about their achievements and success.

Our subconscious cannot differentiate between DOs and DON'Ts. Let's compare two simple commands:

* "DON'T look to your right! Please DON'T!" Where would you look, or where do you want to look?

* "Look to the right! To the right please!" Where would you look?

In both scenarios, you are looking to the right! Your mind just misses that DON'T point, and catches the only bottom line phrase "to the right."

Have you ever seen parents who endlessly tell their children: don't touch, don't run, don't yell, don't eat that, don't interrupt, etc.? The more frequently parents say those things, the less their children listen to them. A child just totally ignores all those DON'Ts. A better strategy is to tell children what to DO. For example "don't run" may be replaced with "sit here for a moment and play with this." Or, for our healthy purpose, the reasonable "Don't eat candy" may be replaced with "Eat this sweet juicy peach."

We need to provide our consciousness with positive DESIRABLE information, and not with something we don't want, don't like, or are afraid of.

Avoid saying, "I don't want to be poor (sick, lonely, fat and ugly, unhappy or broke). Instead say, "I want to be rich (healthy, happily married, slim and good looking, happy and successful)." Do you feel the difference? It is huge!

If you think or say something you actually don't want, you FEEL that way. If you say, "I am SO lonely, no one likes me," you immediately feel worse. Your subconscious mistakenly accepts it as something that you WANT, pictures it and brings it into reality. The results are exactly the opposite and you are getting more and more of something you DO NOT want in your life. However, when you use different words to express your feelings, you also start to THINK positively. The subconscious gets the message and starts drawing the different picture. This time it accepts your message correctly, according to your actual desires. Since it does not know that you are still a little bit far from there, you need to "tilt" it in your favor. This requires some experience, but after consistent practicing you'll become a master at doing so. Don't feel guilty; you are doing it for your better future.

The 5-Step Formula for Managing Negative Thoughts

There are five major steps in this tricky process:

* Awareness, recognition
* Admitting the situation
* Cancellation
* Substitution, replacement
* Letting go

Let's discuss each of these steps in more detail.

AWARENESS is the first step in reprogramming the negative thinking. Before you even plan any actions, you need to be AWARE of your negative thoughts, recognize them, and learn to face them.

For example, start catching yourself using such words and phrases like:

* I can't
* I don't
* I don't want
* I can try
* I need
* I have to
* I must
* I hate

At first glance, they sound innocent, but usually expand into negative sentences and will bring you a whole bouquet of negative feelings.

ADMITTING seems very similar to awareness and is a very short phase in the "catching every thought" process. It plays a bigger role in personal transformation process (which will be described later), but starts from here, from your everyday tiny-mini negative thoughts. Admitting means that you are not only aware that the thought exists, but you're taking responsibility for that; now you know where you are, and are ready to take action.

The CANCELLATION step is easy. Once your thought has been hooked and judged, you just say "Cancel! Cancel!" (out loud if possible) and replace it with a different, more positive, thought. I learned to use this tool at the Silva Method course. This unique Silva technique is dated back to the sixties, and is very effective.

REPLACEMENT. At this point your negative thought is still fresh and sits in your mind; it should be replaced with a positive one as soon as possible. Don't put too much effort into that, just replace it with the opposite word that quickly comes to mind. For example, Hate-Like, Stupid-Smart, Ugly-Cute, Noisy-Quiet, Must-Want, Can't-Can, Try-Do, Don't want-Want etc. Later, you'll become more creative and will easily replace every negative thought with a colorful positive picture. This is a very powerful tool. Remember how our mind pictures our thoughts? Help it, and provide it with a beautiful positive picture! I do it by imagining slides of a presentation. Click - Next please! Instead of a slide showing an empty cold house, there is a new one – bright and colorful full of friends, laughter and fun. Picture it, see it and live it. You feel better, don't you?

Now – LET IT GO. Do whatever you did, get busy, forget about negatives and positives – just live your life and enjoy every moment.

If for any reason a new negative thought crosses your mind, capture it and take immediate action. Apply the five steps described above to EVERY negative thought. You'll see the results very soon.

We may not realize that thoughts are not a result, or reflection of outer world, but vice versa – its cause. "How can I think positively if the reality is so sad?" The answer will be – the reality is basically the same for many people. The economy, the climate, the news, food, prices – are the same for thousands people from the same area. However, one person is optimistic and another one always complains. It happens even in families, where the reality for all family members is the same indeed. The difference is in where WE stand and how WE see ourselves in that reality.

Managing your thoughts is just a habit and an easily learnable skill. When I first read about this process in Personal Development books, I was a little skeptical. I wondered how I could think that I am rich if I can barely survive from paycheck to paycheck. How can I think that I am happy, if I still have not met my soulmate? How can I think that I am full of energy, if I am exhausted and haven't been on a vacation for two years? Concern is reasonable, right? But since all the Self Improvement gurus advised me to do nothing but cancel these negative thoughts, I said I would do that. After all, I had nothing to lose.

I started consciously replacing my negative thoughts with positive ones. If I just couldn't think positively in some cases, at least I did my best not to concentrate and spend too much time on those negative thoughts. This was my small but important first step. At least I didn't think negatively; I wouldn't think about that issue at all. Instead, I would ignore it completely.

So, I started to practice. At the beginning, it was extremely uncomfortable and felt just stupid. I literally FORCED myself to replace my thoughts or ignore them.

My mental process went like this:

* "OMG, he is SO annoying. I can't hear his voice anymore" – "Cancel! Cancel! I believe that there are many people who love him." Hmmm...Still doesn't help. So at least, "Why should I care?"

* "That girl from customer service is so slow!" – "Cancel! She is doing her job; she is tired of talking to so many impatient customers; she has a script to follow and must do that. Calm down."

* "I am tired; I need a treat; I want that cranberry-walnut pie NOW. It will make me happy. "– "Stop it! Cancel! You know this is not true. This is not a treat and it will not make you happier. Conversely, you'll feel guilty and bad physically, emotionally (and even financially!) after eating that. Buy those fresh berries instead and eat them with sour cream. The serving will fill you with vitamins, energy, and positive emotions. Also, it is simply yummy."

❋ "People are going on vacation, relaxing, traveling around the world and I can't even dream about that right now!!!" – "Cancel! Cancel! You are on a mission and can't spend your time and money on vacations. You'll do it in the future. Look at the beautiful place where you live. You have a beautiful green backyard with all these cute little creatures: squirrels, rabbits, groundhogs and chipmunks. Relax and enjoy the breeze."

Well, I am glad if you are laughing now, because this is also a very positive thing! Usually, we do not control thousands of our daily thoughts; we just think them, that's it. However, controlling your thoughts may even become an interesting journey. Now that you are aware of the process, imagine you are out fishing. When you start catching thoughts, you'll throw away the negative ones, while letting the positive ones grow freely in the ocean of your emotions. Please do your best in practicing this method because it really works!

Gratitude

An additional weapon in fighting negative thoughts is the feeling of Gratitude.

I know that you're probably saying, "How can I be grateful for being fat and lonely? For all those bills I get? For a job I hate and can't quit? No way!"

Believe me, I hear you. I was there; I know your thoughts and feelings. But are you losing anything by just doing this without arguing (no tries, you remember that)? If it helps (and it does!) you'll improve your life. If not, you haven't lost anything. You'll still have everything you have now. Worth doing, isn't it?

So, here you go:

* These f-ing bills keep coming at me! Looks like there is only one address for them on the entire planet! I can't handle them anymore! I hate them! Get out of my life!"

- "Cancel! Thank you! (OK, in this case you might need to repeat it several times out loud just to be sure: Thank you! Thank you! Thank you! Thank you! Hmm…Twice as loud: THANK YOU! THANK YOU! THANK YOU!

Feel a little better? I told you!

- They come to this address because I have a place to live. I have hot water every day; I have a car, and I went out last month with my friends. Thanks for everything I have and for the fact that I am still able to pay for all that. Thank you! Thank you! Thank you!"

You see? It wasn't hard. You did it, and I am proud of you!

I admit that it is much easier to be grateful for something you already have. That's obvious, so it's not worth discussing. The point is that you can always find something to be grateful for. Just think more about that and don't miss a chance to express your appreciation for everything in your life. When you practice that, you'll start to notice how many great things you have. More than that, you'll start noticing something you never paid attention to before! And better things will start appearing in your life as a RESULT of your appreciation. Believe me, this is true.

Frequently I hear "Yep…it makes sense, but life is too complicated and it is easier to say…" Basically it is not. It's the opposite. Life is easier than we think it is. To DO is easier than to say. Our thoughts are full of UNREASONABLE fears and doubts. However, when you know exactly what you want, life itself gives you an answer. You just need to keep your final goal in mind and move toward it. Then, when you do it and it's over, you will say "Ha! It was easy!" I am sure you have many examples like that from your own experience.

However, even the most optimistic people are sometimes emotionally down, think negatively and express their negative feelings. It's normal; we are human. That is the point. We ARE human. Therefore, we have a GIFT to CONTROL our thoughts and manage our lives. No one can do it for you better than you can. You and only you know your deep inner dreams, your desires, and your mission. And there is only one person in the entire Universe who can make it a reality – YOU.

By controlling your thoughts, you clear your subconscious mind from everything that keeps you back. Imagine your subconscious mind as a beautiful garden; you definitely don't want to see any ugly weeds growing there, do you? So, weed the garden of your thoughts, take a good care of it and it will bring you gorgeous fruits of happiness, health and prosperity.

"You are today where your thoughts have brought you;
You will be tomorrow where your thoughts take you."
James Allen

Replacing Thoughts about Food

When I practiced medicine in Israel, as it usually happens in women's groups, over lunch we talked about families, cooking and eating. There is a specific Russian cuisine dish called "borscht." Originally, a Ukrainian ethnic food, it may be described as a rich flavored stew, made of beef, potatoes, cabbage, beets, carrots, tomato paste and spices. It is delicious and very popular among the Russian speaking population and also in some European countries. One of the nurses was from Poland; she knew about borscht and asked me once if I cook it. "Yes," I replied, "We like borscht, but it's too hot now, we only cook it in the winter." She was laughing hysterically and said aloud, "You see? That's why she is thin! Her THOUGHTS are thin! She thinks that borscht is good only for the winter. For us it's ALWAYS good!!!" Honestly, at the time I did not get the deep meaning of that statement. Now I understand how smart it is! This is the key! Our thoughts! How we think – so we behave, work, eat, love and live.

Let's analyze some thoughts related to food and eating.

For example:

* This product will expire in two days; we have to eat it today. Don't throw it away.

Honestly, I don't like to discard food, and almost never do. However, if you catch yourself eating something not because you are hungry or because it is delicious, but just because "you have to," fight this habit as soon as possible. At first glance, it is not easy. However, when you overcome your negative thinking and behavioral habits, you'll be on the way to your goal of living a healthy and joyful life.

First, fight the habit of eating after you are already full or to "save" the food. You can throw it away! It sounds ridiculous. You say that, "I'd better throw that food inside of me and hurt my body rather than throw it out." It really does not make any sense. Eating that food IS equal to throwing it out.

If you are about to eat something late at night just because you don't want to put it back in the refrigerator, stop and think for a minute. Use a "procrastination" technique. Place your food in a container and eat it (not now!) – but tomorrow for lunch. This strategy has several benefits. First, you will not eat late at night. Second, you will not be throwing away still good food. And third, you don't need to buy your lunch tomorrow since you already have it, so you will save money. And the most important thing is that you will be taking the first step in eliminating your previous bad habits.

* This casserole is not tasty and too fatty, but I am embarrassed to leave it on the plate.

No one can force you to eat something that isn't tasty or unhealthy at the party or in the restaurant. Sometimes you think that not eating means you're not polite or you're hurting someone's feelings. In reality, this is not the case. Have you ever noticed what or how much other people eat at the party? I really don't think so, unless you watch other people very closely. Even so, most likely you have a better reason for watching someone other than what he or she is eating. The same goes for them. Someone probably can't take his or her eyes off of YOU, but not because of the FOOD on your plate. So, please don't even bother thinking whether other people are watching what you eat—they're simply NOT watching your food intake!

Declarations:

- *I focus on positive over negative, on opportunities over obstacles*

- *I think only healthy thoughts that empower me*

- *My thoughts take me to my destiny*

The Recipe of the Chapter:

Country Style Oatmeal Crepes

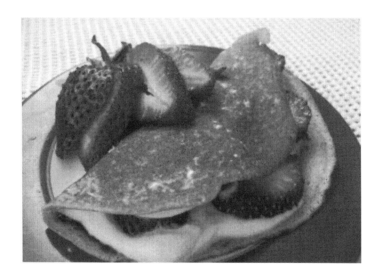

Oatmeal flour itself has a medium GI of 40. However, since it is a carbohydrate, you shouldn't eat these crepes with products that have fat, such as butter, sour cream or whipped cream. Such high GI carbohydrates as honey, maple (or any other) syrup or regular jams shouldn't be used either. The healthy way of eating these crepes is with 0% Greek yogurt and/or 100% fruit jam. All kinds of fresh fruits and berries can be also freely added to the breakfast. Please carefully follow the idea of product combinations. Using even a 2% yogurt is not recommended and may cause you to gain weight.

Ingredients:
½ cup of dry milk
2 cups of water
1/3 cup of olive oil
2 eggs
2 cups of oatmeal flour
2 tablespoons spelt flour
½ teaspoon baking powder
2 teaspoons fructose or Splenda
2 dashes of salt

Mix all the ingredients in a medium bowl and beat well until combined. The batter may look too liquid, but oatmeal flour will swell. Leave the batter at room temperature for several hours. I like making it in the evening, so in the morning it is ready for cooking. Beat the mixture again before cooking. Add some more flour or water, if needed. Cook crepes in a small Teflon frying pan over high heat, about 1 minute on each side, or until they are golden brown. Since you're using olive oil in the batter mixture, the crepes will not stick to the pan. However, I recommend putting a little bit of olive oil in the frying pan before cooking the first crepe.

This is a great cozy breakfast for everyone in the family; it is healthy and delicious!

Chapter 6 : Goal Setting

"People with goals succeed because they know where they're going"
Earl Nightingale

We often hear that goal setting is important to succeed in life. Why do we need to set goals at all? How should we be setting them to ensure that we make them work?

If you don't set up your trip destination, how can you get there? You can't. You'll be going around again, and again and then come back exhausted and disappointed. Then you'll say, "Setting goals doesn't work!" What doesn't work is NOT setting a goal, or setting it incorrectly.

Where do our goals come from? From our DESIRE. When you know exactly WHAT you want, you are more likely to set your goals and find a way to achieve them. Recall the Process of Manifestation formula:

Past Programming→Thoughts→Feelings→Actions→**Results**

Now, the goal comes between Feelings and Actions, and definitely influences our results. Therefore, the newly revised formula will be:

Past Programming→Thoughts→Feelings→**GOALS**→
Actions→**Results**

Goals take an important place there, and cannot be ignored under any circumstances.

Setting goals correctly helps us and influences our performance in several ways:

* Allows us to focus on the relevant tasks
* Enables us to keep the commitment
* Helps us develop learning strategies

They also

* Keep us motivated
* Influence our success oriented behavior

In terms of reaching a healthy lifestyle, goal setting would focus on how you can achieve your ideal weight.

Firstly, always think about "reducing" weight, not "losing" it. When you **lose** something, you can find it again one day.

However, getting rid of your extra pounds is not an instance of wanting to find them in the future. Your purpose is to lose them forever and never "find" them again.

How to set your goal to achieve the results you want

Timing is everything. To make your goal work, you need to choose a correct time for that. When does the average person make a decision to start a diet? Usually it happens when you suddenly look in the mirror and are shocked to see the extra pounds everywhere. "OMG! I am a pig! I am so fat and ugly!" Then you immediately make a decision to start a diet. "Enough is enough!"- You say bravely, "I start dieting right NOW!" However, this is a big mistake. The timing is off and not suitable for setting a goal.

Why is it important? Believe it or not, during your goal achievement process, you'll frequently go back to that basic point. Do you want to go back to a statement such as "I am ugly and I hate myself?" Definitely not. If you do, it will distract you and instead of pushing you forward, it will hold you back. Then one day, you'll be tired of your diet, weary of being hungry, and sick of your omnipresent "I am ugly and I hate myself" statement.

Then you will look at yourself and think, "Hmm...Not too bad...I think I lost a couple of pounds...I am still OK." That's it. Your diet will be over, because you established your goal at the wrong moment, when you were thinking negatively about yourself, rather than positively.

Click the 'Undo' button now. Let's go back to your mirror. Now look at yourself again and ADMIT the things that you don't like - ALL OF THEM. Do not lie to yourself. It's important that you're honest. Don't be afraid or embarrassed. There are no witnesses here. Do it. Say it OUT LOUD and then write it down. Write down everything you hate about yourself, everything you see and FEEL. This is not about the number; this is about your FEELINGS regarding that number. This is not about counting; this is about disengagement and growing.

It's also a perfect time to enhance all your fears. If you smoke and can't quit, picture your lungs full of nicotine, and your fear of getting lung cancer. If you are obese, do you want to die suddenly on the street from a cardiovascular attack, or end up paralyzed after suffering a stroke? Do you want to suffer from diabetes and end up with vision problems and skin wounds? All those things happen to thousands of people every year, and may happen to you - if you ignore your weight and don't take care of yourself.

You may not like this step, but it is a necessary part of overcoming those bad feelings. Don't think, "I am still OK" because you're still healthy, and "I am not TOO ugly. After all, other people are worse off, and in fact, I am pretty." You certainly are, but hold off on the self-compliments; you'll have time for them later. Now it's time for you to be critical and judgmental. Yes, it requires courage. Be your own doctor, psychotherapist and judge.

Unfortunately, most people prefer to AVOID the situation. Almost everyone avoids discussing money issues or their relationship woes. They avoid admitting their extra pounds and bad health. But you are different. You are reading this book and want to improve your life. If you find yourself in a hole, – stop digging! ADMIT IT!!!! Avoiding doesn't accomplish anything. Admitting will rescue you.

Do not make any decisions at this point; do not set any goals. This is not the starting point for transformation; this is the first step IN transformation. There is no future success without this step. Without admitting, there is no canceling (you have nothing to cancel) and there is no replacement (you have nothing to replace). It means that without admitting, your life will stay the same. Admitting is your new BEGINNING.

Once you are ready for the next step, you need a positive start for your goal. Now it's time to set the goal. Think about being healthy and beautiful, sexy and energetic, about being a great example for your kids, loved ones, family, friends and everyone around you.

Once you decide to go for it, take responsibility for your decision and don't give up! If your family and friends support you, you can make a public commitment. Sharing your goal will help you to keep your promise. Also, it will make the people around you proud when you achieve it. Having someone else on your side and moving forward together is an even better idea. It turns that lonely process into an adventure and guarantees better results.

Have a clear idea in mind. Thinking something like "It would be good to lose (!) several pounds by Christmas" doesn't help and doesn't work. Your real goal should be:

* Clear
* Specific and measurable
* Challenging, but realistic and achievable
* Stated in a present tense rather than in a future tense

Think about a certain number of pounds by which you can reduce your weight over a certain period of time. Promising yourself to be 10 pound less by next week is obviously a promise to fail and would also be dangerous to your health.

Write your goals down and make them visible. Buy a fancy piece of paper (you and your goal deserve it!), put you goal there and sign it.

For example:

I, _____(your name),

weigh ....(lb) by...... .(month/day/year).

Today's date and your signature_____

Put it on the refrigerator or on the wall where you can see it during the day.

Break your big goal into several smaller goals. Losing 3 pounds a month may not sound too exciting; however it means reducing 36 pounds per year! This is a great achievement with a healthy and balanced approach. Also, the chances that you'll be able to keep that weight off are good.

Celebrate each of your achievements (please, not with cheesecake!). Maybe buying new clothes after reducing the first couple of pounds is too soon, but buying a new belt will increase your desire to continue, and remind you about your small victory.

Immediately get rid of clothes that are too big for you! Remember, since you are not going to "find" your weight again, you don't need them anymore. As soon as you become one size smaller, take those big clothes out of your closet. Donate them, throw them away, even burn and dance around them, but never keep them. Be excited about buying new clothes in the future; you will need them and you'll enjoy shopping!

I would also like to highlight the importance of imagination in the goals achievement process. I have no doubts that you are a responsible and strong person, and ready to achieve your goal whatever it takes. However, willpower is not enough, not just for you, but for everyone. It's not that I'm a pessimistic and negative person (otherwise I would never write this book), but the truth is that **it is almost impossible to change habits using only willpower.** We all need the spice of imagination to make it work.

As I've stressed, the basic starting point should be positive. Focusing on dieting and avoiding fattening foods makes you think about the problem, not the solution. This is negative thinking, because you are focusing on what you DON'T want - losing the food you have always liked. This will not take you far. Instead, you need to focus on what you WANT, on your NEW desire, new behavior, and on your new CHOICE.

What do you want instead of bad food habits and being overweight? How will you profit from achieving your ideal weight? Think about all the benefits you can enjoy by materializing that goal:

* Better health (lower sugar and cholesterol level if this is a problem now)

* Being lighter

* Having more energy without consuming energy drinks

* Being sexier

* Setting a great example for your loved ones

* Having more self esteem

* Being more satisfied with life

* Appearing more attractive and elegant

* Finding a soulmate

* Attracting more customers

* Making more sales

* Earning more money

❋ Buying better clothes

❋ Traveling around the world

You see? Is it just about your weight? No, it's about your whole LIFE! Feel free to expand the list; it's about YOUR life.

> *"If you want to reach a goal,*
> *you must "see the reaching" in your own mind*
> *before you actually arrive at your goal"*
> *Zig Ziglar*

A good way to overcome a negative habit and move toward your desired life is to imagine yourself already DOING that and experiencing the feelings associated with it. Experience it completely as if it has already happened. Live the life of your dreams NOW. Visualize yourself being a smaller size, and feeling elegant and attractive. Imagine how you FEEL buying new clothes, FEEL how they touch your elegant body. Imagine choosing new styles and colors. Imagine how other people are looking at you and enjoy it! Remember these feelings and let them inspire you.

Some people say "Affirmations don't work!" They obviously don't bring what's desired after we repeat them 300 times, or even 3000 times. This is not how they work. Their job is to direct our THINKING. They help us put positive SEEDS of success in our subconscious mind slowly, but deeply. The results may be invisible for a long time, and this is when many people quit. If you repeat "I am rich and healthy" without doing anything, you are definitely not getting a million dollar check by mail and you won't wake up weighing 20 pound less the next morning. However, day after day, you will start THINKING differently without even noticing that. Since you THINK differently, you start to ACT differently. Your new ACTIONS will bring you new RESULTS. Later, when you naturally choose a 'Salmon with asparagus' over 'Double cheeseburger with fries,' you will have the affirmations credit! YOU did it, and the affirmations you repeated helped you.

> *"People often say that motivation doesn't last.*
> *Well, neither does bathing — that's why we*
> *recommend it daily."*
> *Zig Ziglar*

In order for affirmations to succeed, you must BELIEVE in what you say and FEEL it. The more positive you think and FEEL about your desire, the more appropriately you ACT, and those actions will make that dream your reality.

Know that you have made an important life changing decision. By achieving your goals of getting healthier, you are changing a great deal of other important things in your life.

How can we manage our feelings and stay focused on the goals we set? The answer is simple--choose the right thoughts. Just as you had to replace your negative thoughts about bills, job or circumstances, you can practice replacing thoughts about food. For example:

Thought 1: I desire to be healthy, beautiful and in good shape.

Goal: Reduce 40 pounds in 1 year, weigh 120 pounds, keep this weight forever in the future.

Action 1: Weekly sessions with a personal coach, changing the Eating Blueprint, creating the everyday menu from only the recommended products.

* Though 2: I want this cake NOW….

* Cancel! This thought does not match your Goal! It should be replaced with another one, more positive and suitable for your Goal.

* Thought 3: I'd better eat dried fruits with nuts. They are really delicious and much healthier.

* Action 2: Eating dry fruits with nuts, according to Thought 3 and not Thought 2.

Result: Reducing 40 pounds in a year, achieving your ideal weight of 120 pounds.

Reward: Feeling light and increasing the energy level, satisfied and proud of yourself, buying new fancy clothes, compliments of friends and colleagues, enhancing your self-esteem, promotion and work, making more money and having more excited things in your life!

Think about what you think. Taste every one of your thoughts. What do they taste like? Are you feeling cheered up and more confident or do they bring you weakness and excuses? Make your choice in favor of those which take you closer to your desire. Little by little, you'll think beneficial thoughts subconsciously, without any effort. By then you'll forget about extra pounds and worries about gaining them ever again. Since you will understand how easy and how effectively you can manage your nutrition, you just won't be able to eat something that hurts you. Eating gourmet food without gaining weight? I think everyone would love this! When you know WHAT you want, filled with enthusiasm and acting accordingly, there is no doubt of your success. Therefore, the only thing you need now is your WISH to be healthy and happy!

"No one is in your way – just YOU"
Paulo Coelho

Declarations:

- *I know what I want and I go for it*

- *I set my goals wisely*

- *I taste my thoughts to achieve my goals*

ᏮᎢᎷᎥᎧ

The Recipe of the Chapter:

Piquant Meat-Stuffed Artichoke Bottoms

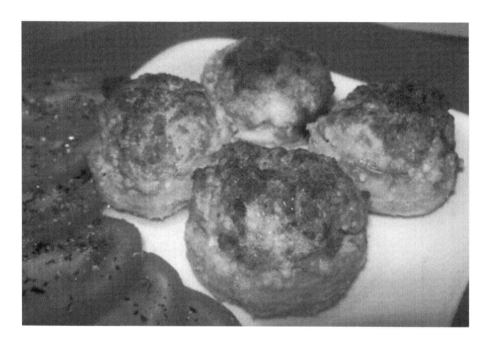

Artichokes are part of the Fiber food category and their GI is only 15. They can be healthily combined with lipids and proteins. This meal is delicious and flavorful, and the cooking is easy and quick.

2 cans (14 oz. each) of artichoke bottoms

For stuffing:
1 grated onion
½ pound ground beef
½ pound ground chicken
½ pound of ground turkey
2 teaspoons of Worcestershire sauce
Salt and black pepper
Grated Parmesan

Mix all the ingredients. Place 1-2 tablespoons of the stuffing in each artichoke bottom (or more, if they are big). Now scoop up the grated Parmesan into your palm, then dip and roll the meat side of the stuffed artichoke in it. The parmesan won't melt while cooking. It will shape the stuffing and will create a golden crust.

Place the stuffed artichoke bottoms in a baking dish and cook them in a 430*F oven for 25-30 minutes.

Chapter 7 : Your Super Self

"It's not the size of the dog in the fight; it is the size of the fight in the dog"
Mark Twain

I was considering making this chapter the first chapter of this book, but then decided to place it after the Goals chapter, in order to support, inspire and encourage you.

I want you to understand that building a relationship with yourself must happen before you're able to build relationships with others, and this step is critical for your success. Do you remember reading that our outer world is a reflection of our inner world? It is very important to become and BE a "worthy" person to find the right people. You must put yourself first, and then you will attract the right people.

In everyday life, we usually use a term - 'Self Esteem.' We may say that someone has high self-esteem, and that's why he or she is happily married, or that his self-esteem is low, so that is why he got involved with the wrong person. You see, even not knowing about 'inner world-outer world' correlation, we picture that correctly.

In fact, Self Esteem is only one component of your Super Self. There are two other factors: Self Image and Self Confidence.

* Self Image describes what we THINK about ourselves
* Self Esteem describes what we FEEL about ourselves
* Self Confidence is how we ACT

Combine them together and we are back to the Process of Manifestation formula again!

Thought + Feelings +Actions = Results

Thoughts, Feelings and Actions are our Inner world, our Super Self. The more SUPER we think, feel and act, the more SUPER our results.

What is the taste of your thoughts?

* Health and happiness, or fear of diseases and failure?
* Joy, or suffering?
* Abundance, or fear of poverty?
* Happy relationships, or "It is not for me, I am not worthy"

Your thoughts are your initial steps to your Super Self. When you think about health, joy, abundance and happiness, you FEEL that way. You feel that way – you ACT that way. They are your tiny but strong bricks in building your reality.

In discussing your Super Self, we are back again to the Blueprint point. Do you love yourself or not? Are you proud of yourself, or feel guilty? Are you the best, or not worthy?

Whatever answer you have, it comes from your Blueprint. The roots are the same: family, babysitters, nanny, teachers, friends, acquaintance, social media, religion, traditions or any personal experience in the past. If during your childhood, you heard phrases such as "Good girl/ boy!" "Great job!" "You can do that!" "You are the best!" "I am proud of you!" – Your self-esteem is likely high and healthy. Unfortunately, not everyone is lucky enough to hear those sweet comments during the childhood. Even if your family wasn't cruel, some families may be just very cold in expressing emotions. Your parents might love you unconditionally, but were unable to tell you they did. Other parents might think that expressing love is indulgent and their children may grow up to be too selfish. Many parents and teachers never pay attention to achievements, but instead highlight every failure.

Another scenario occurs when a child is loved and supported by his or her family, but is very shy and thinks that he or she is "not worthy." This feeling may come from a tiny episode in the past, when someone—perhaps even a stranger—said something that deeply hurt the child. The person may not even remember what was said but will remember the FEELING, and that feeling may influence his or her entire life.

Often, when someone told us something in the past, it was automatically accepted as a correct claim. We just sponged the statement without filtering. Anyone could call you a 'piggy,' or if your parents were angry at you for a moment and called you 'stupid'' or someone rejected your offer to have lunch together. We carry that incident or comment with us for years and behave according to those hurtful words.

Now think for a moment – what if that person wasn't right? You were just told something is obviously WRONG. Why should the other person's wrong idea or words or actions influence YOUR life? The fact that you've heard something doesn't mean that you should accept that! Literally, you have nothing to deal with! Ignore it and move forward!

As kids, we definitely cannot do that. We don't have our own life experience yet; we depend on adults. We "should listen" to them and be "good kids." However, you don't have to carry those other-people-ideas through your entire life. This is called **"playing the victim"**. Do you like to pity yourself? I admit that in certain circumstances we all like doing that. "Oh, I am a poor little soul..." The question is "How long does it take you?" If you do it constantly on a regular basis and for a long time, you are wasting your life. Be aware of what you're doing and take action. That should be treated by YOU. *

If these feelings last a day or two once a year, there's nothing wrong, and this emotion may even help as a stress release. If you feel discouraged, decide that you will allow yourself

---

* We are not talking about medical conditions which can cause those feelings. This is not the purpose of this book and not the area of my expertise. If you feel too anxious and depressed about yourself, you should probably consider talking to a medical professional.

to feel that way! Get crazy, cry, eat and drink whatever you want, go deeper and deeper into that emotion, FEEL your pity and enjoy the feeling! Then, take a piece of paper and write down all your thoughts about how bad "those people" are, what a "poor little soul you are," and how badly you feel about that. Take more paper (and more tissue) if one sheet is not enough to express everything you feel. You are not going to share that with the rest of the world, so don't be shy. By doing that, you TREAT yourself. After you are done - BURN it! If you have a fireplace, do it there. If not, find another safe place where you can destroy all the papers. Then, take another sheet of paper and write down how you want it to be YOUR way. I wouldn't recommend writing about how you want other people to behave; you are not influencing THEM. Just write down how you want to see the situation.

For example, your paper might state, "My boss drives me crazy! He controls everything I do; he watches me closely, and wants everything his way. He is not open-minded and is very annoying! I hate it! I hate my job!!! Poor-poor-poor me…"

Please don't write something like, "I want him to come to me and apologize, take me off all my projects and double my salary." I agree it sounds very tempting, but that means you're writing about him, not about YOU.

Instead write: "I want to do what I love. It is great to enjoy my job and have good relationships with my colleagues. I would like to get well paid for my contributions. I'll be happy to love my job!"

Respond this way to every point of your anger and disappointments. Write down how you wish it, what would make you happy, and think about circumstances, people and yourself. Keep your notes.

I have found this technique to be very helpful and powerful. Before building a new desire, we need to completely destroy our doubts to ourselves and complaints towards other people. Stay in it for a little bit, FEEL it, and remember those feelings. It will help you stop playing the victim. Briefly pity yourself to build your new, DESIRED reality.

There are not many options here. Actually, you have only two choices:

1. Continue playing the victim and stay there for the rest of your life

2. Stop playing the victim, move forward, and CREATE your life according to YOUR template.

Which one sounds better to you? In this case, you cannot have both. There is no such thing as a "happy victim." If you pity yourself and blame others for everything that happens to you, you block your road to success. By success, I mean ANY success, from a small personal achievement to global international fame, if you wish to be there.

> *"The most creative act you will ever undertake is the act of creating yourself"*
> *Deepak Chopra, M.D.*

Do Not Compare

This is one of the main principles of Self Development. You don't need to BE better than anyone else. You don't need to DO better than anyone else. You are a worthwhile person just as you are.

First, how do you know that "they are better"? If someone is slimmer, cuter, richer, or more famous, it doesn't mean that person is better than you. It just means that he or she weighs less, has a smaller nose (blond/ black/ orange hair, green/ blue/ black eyes) has more money and is more well known. That's it. He or she can be a great person too, but it doesn't mean that he or she is BETTER than you. They are just different people. Just because they may be good, why does that make you not worthy? There is enough space for many great people on the planet. There's no reason for you to give up and voluntarily enroll yourself in a "not worthy" population.

There is an old and slightly naughty joke that fits this topic:

A gentleman comes to the doctor and says, "Doctor, I am getting sexually weak. I can't make love every night anymore"

Doctor asks, "And how frequently can you make it?"

"Twice a week I am fine"

Doctor replies, "But Mr. Johnson, you are 70 years old; this is great for your age!"

"I can't agree, doctor. My neighbor is age 75 and does it 5 times a day"

"How do you know?"

"He told me!"

"Well then… you tell him the same thing."

This is about the "THEY" syndrome. We are too involved in comparing ourselves to THEM.

* They told me
* They know better
* They are not interested
* They are well educated
* They are lucky
* They got better genes than me
* They are from a wealthy family
* They have spouses/kids/parents/pets
* They own a house/boat/BMW/business
* They are smart/rich/happy

I always ask, "Who are THEY?" and then back to the question "How do you know?"

Listen to what I'm saying. I am not telling you that THEY DON'T. There are always, ALWAYS people around you who are smarter, younger, healthier, cuter, slimmer, richer, better educated and "luckier." So what? If you spend the rest of your life trying to compete with them and pitying yourself, it will not make you THEM anyway. Do not aim to be like them. Think about being the smarter, healthier and younger looking, cuter, slimmer, richer, better educated, luckier and happier YOU. Everyone has their own uniqueness and you should aim to develop that, become the even better YOU and then share that with people.

Another syndrome that may hold us back is the "IF" syndrome.

* How can I be happy? I am so fat! IF I lose weight, I'll be much happier!

* IF only I had a decent job, my life would be different!

* IF only I meet a nice guy/girl, it will motivate me to lose weight.

* IF only I had a lot of money, I would invest it wisely.

You get the point. What happens here, is switching the reason with a result.

Reduce your weight, find a decent job, learn how to manage whatever money you have, and you WILL feel happy, meet a nice guy/girl, and become rich. Don't think IF – think WHEN.

"Do what you can, with what you have, where you are"
Theodore Roosevelt

Another syndrome similar to the IF syndrome is the BUT syndrome:

* I would like to start my own business, BUT I don't have any initial money and need to learn marketing

* I'll be happy to eat healthy, BUT my family does not accept this food

* I want to go to that party, BUT I have nothing to wear

* I would apply for that program, BUT my scores are not excellent and THEY will not accept me (oh-oh! we even got "two for the price of one" here!)

Those BUTs are destroying all our efforts from the very beginning. Even if we were thinking about making any progress, after those "BUT" thoughts, we end up losing our enthusiasm completely. What kind of Feelings can we develop thinking like this? What kind of Actions can we take? So there are no Results either.

Now, would you please replace those BUTs with ANDs? Take your time.

Do you see what happens? When you do so, the sentences sound differently. They don't destroy your initial idea anymore, they sound as if you are beginning a new project. They call you to take actions! You will want to find answers on where to earn more money and learn marketing, how to introduce your family to a new food, how to get well dressed for the party you wish to go to, and what to do to be accepted to the desired program. The small effort you make toward replacing just one word can help you change your world.

Self-Love or Selfishness?

It may be confusing to understand the difference between Loving Yourself and being Selfish, especially for women, who are accustomed to caring for their families. Women often forget themselves as they focus on doing their best for their husband, children, parents and extended family. These women don't have time to love themselves. Sometimes, a woman even believes that this behavior isn't right. She may wonder how she can put herself first. What kind of mother and wife will I be if I do so?! Right? Wrong.

Loving yourself means doing what YOU want, investing in your physical and mental health, growing your positive emotions and becoming a better person. If you don't put an oxygen mask on yourself first, you will quickly die and you wouldn't be able to help others. If you help yourself first – you'll stay alive and help many other people. If you don't take care of yourself, you can't take care of your husband, children, parents and extended family. Self-Love is a win-win scenario.

Being Selfish means wanting OTHER people to do what YOU want. Perhaps you're thinking:

* ❋ I want to go to the party; YOU HAVE TO buy me a new dress.

* I don't have money for a babysitter; THEY HAVE TO help me take care of my kids

* IF you don't listen to me and don't do what I say, I will not make a Birthday Party for you.

This is called being selfish, manipulating, and forcing people to behave YOUR way.

And this is not in anyone's favor. This is egotistical and silly. Even if they do, it cannot last very long. Selfishness is a lose-lose situation, and you are not that kind of person anyway.

Success Journal

Have you ever thought about keeping a success journal? If you did, do you have it? Are you documenting and keeping track of your achievements on a daily basis? If you haven't done so yet, this is a perfect time to start.

Purchase a fancy journal. Choose your favorite color, favorite shape and appealing textured cover. You will be using it daily, so you should love the journal and enjoy holding it in your hands.

Every night, before going to bed, write down the date and list your five key achievements for that day. It does not matter how big they are. Perhaps, you started applying for a postgraduate degree, or simply sent an email to a friend. The important thing is to honor yourself, to recognize those tiny but important paces in your Self Growing process.

If you have a clear goal in mind, coordinate your achievements with your goal. For example, if you are working on reducing your weight, concentrate on those achievements first:

1. I've read the article about five healthy foods

2. I ate grilled chicken and fresh salad for dinner

3. I did not eat donuts offered at the staff meeting this morning

4. I took a half-hour walk in the evening

5. I cooked whole grain pasta with vegetables for tomorrow's lunch.

Sometimes you don't have five achievements related to your goal. In that case, start with related achievements and add any other unrelated ones. They are still yours, so give yourself some credit:

1. I ate whole grain pasta with vegetables for lunch.

2. I declined to go out for pizza, so I ate healthier food and saved money

3. I took my kids out for an evening walk, and we had a great time together

4. I finally called my mother-in-law, and even stayed calm during that conversation

5. I've read *Men Are from Mars Women Are from Venus* by John Gray, to improve my relationships

You'll be amazed how keeping a journal will motivate you and influence your Super Self positively! You will start noticing positive things about yourself, you'll start appreciating the great moments in your life, and you'll do much more every day. Since you know that you MUST have a daily achievement for your journal, you will DO many more great things! Read your notes periodically. Remind yourself how great you are, and how many great things you do every single day.

Actually, there is only one person with whom you need to compare yourself. It's YOU. Compare today's YOU with yesterday's YOU. Did you make progress during the day? Week? Month or year? Write down all your achievements and celebrate the victories. Then, establish a new goal, raising the bar higher and do your best to achieve that. Then, analyze your success and (yes!) compare yourself with... YOURSELF. Be proud of your achievements and be willing to achieve more. It will stimulate you, inspire you and will help you succeed. Since only YOU can do it for yourself, don't wait. Start NOW.

Only You

No one on Earth
Exists quite like you
And no one is able
To do what you do

The person you are
The talents you bear
Gifts that only
You can share

Only you have learned
From the things you've done
Gaining perspective
From the battles you've won

Times when you've lost
Have been priceless too
The lessons contribute
To what makes you You

The rest of the world
Can't see through your eyes
Which is why your insight
Is such a prize.

** The *Only You* poem is a copyrighted excerpt from the book *The Elusive Here & Now* by Dan Coppersmith. It is reprinted here with permission from the author. www.SpiritWire.com

Because you are you
There are lives you affect
Much more than you
Would ever expect

The things you do
The things you say
Send ripples throughout
The Milky Way

You're unique, amazing
Like no one else
You have the exclusive
On being yourself.

Dan Coppersmith

Declarations:

- *I am bigger than any problem, I can easily handle anything*

- *There are so many things that make me special*

- *I am good enough just the way I am*

The Recipe of the Chapter:

My special bonus for SUPER YOU is two Recipes
in this chapter!

Extravagant Three Layer Salad

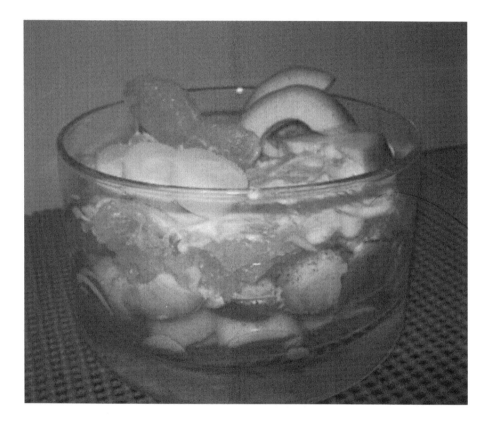

2 pink grapefruits
2 avocados
1 can of palm hearts
3 tablespoons of real mayonnaise without added sugar or
starch
1 teaspoon of ketchup

Salt and pepper
A little bit of lemon juice to sprinkle on avocados

Remove skin from grapefruit and divide them into segments.
Remove skin from each segment and cut them into 3-4 pieces
Cut avocados and palm hearts into ½ inch pieces
Mix mayonnaise with ketchup

Take a crystal dish and place the ingredients in layers:

* Palm hearts on the bottom, sprinkle with salt and pepper
* Add 1 tablespoon of the mayonnaise-ketchup mix
* Place the avocados as a second layer; sprinkle them with lemon, salt and pepper
* Add 1 tablespoon of the mayonnaise-ketchup mix
* Add grapefruit as a third layer
* The rest of the mayonnaise-ketchup mix goes on the top

I recommend keeping a couple of extra avocado slices and grapefruit lobes for decoration.

This salad should be prepared immediately before serving. However, you can prepare grapefruits one day before, and keep them in a container in the refrigerator. When you start making the salad, get rid of all the juice.

The GI is low, the components are healthy, and their combination is tasty and appealing!

Light Pineapple Cocktail

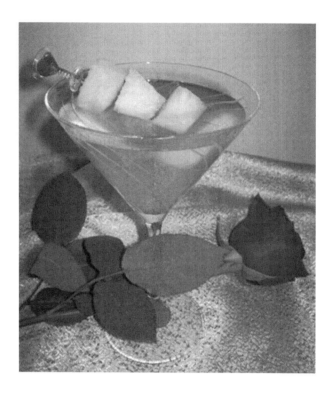

* 2 parts gin
* 2 parts dry vermouth
* 4 parts pineapple juice
* 16 drops of Aromatic Bitters
* Mint
* Pineapple slices and mint leaves for decoration

Put all the ingredients into a cocktail shaker filled with ice. Shake and drain into a martini glass. Garnish with pineapple slices and mint leaves.

Chapter 8 : To Your Success

"Ask and you shall receive, seek and you shall find, knock and it shall be opened unto you."

Matthew 7:7

*T*he truth is that there are many roadblocks in rebuilding the Eating Blueprint and creating a new lifestyle. However, every effort and every tiny step count, because by acting consistently you invest in creating a HABIT.

It's comparable with developing a habit of managing money. Some people work hard and earn a solid salary, but they're still in debt and have no savings. Usually, these people say that life is short; they work hard and deserve to keep spending. They may want to travel, and since they'll never save enough, why shouldn't they take out another loan so they can live NOW. This behavior may make sense, but never for the long term. The point is that NOW they are NOT living the life they want. Instead of avoiding unnecessary spending and investing wisely, they spend everything, choosing to pay high interest on credit cards and loans for ambiguous pleasure. Years later, they find themselves even in deeper debt.

On the other hand, by avoiding unnecessary spending in the beginning, saving and investing wisely, they could be financially free NOW. It would require some restrictions and even inconvenience, but with willpower and consistent behavior, it would change their lives for the better, bringing them financial freedom sooner.

When we make a decision to save, it doesn't mean that we will never buy a luxury item for the rest of our life. In fact, when managing money wisely becomes a habit, just the opposite is likely to happen.

By spending everything now, we'll stay in debt and will not be able to have luxuries. But stopping ourselves from spending will allow us to enjoy luxuries later in life. We'll buy them as a reward for our wise savings and investing choices, and will therefore enjoy them even more.

The situation with your health is quite similar. If you continue your bad eating habits, you'll be stuck with them forever. You will go from one low calorie diet to another, from the previous "Before and After" results to the next ones. You'll continue gaining weight, and possibly suffering from diseases. You'll keep eating fries, sandwiches and hamburgers, while refusing to go to a luxury restaurant to enjoy escargots, gorgeous steak or yummy pasta, and unbelievably fancy desserts—all of which may be served in smaller portions and taste much better than the "fast food." However, when you develop new healthy eating habits so deeply that they are "in your mind, heart, blood and soul", you will improve your entire life. You will make the right choices on an everyday basis, build a healthy body, and THEN you can indulge yourself on occasion at a fancy restaurant. As a reward for your everyday wise choices, for taking good care of your body and your health, you'll enjoy your life more. You will be able to have the occasional fancy food but you'll be in peace and balance with yourself.

"We are what we repeatedly do. Excellence, therefore, is not an act, but a habit."

Aristotle

At this point you may be wondering, "How will my life may be happier if I don't eat my favorite cookies anymore?! I like them so much and I need them!"

My first answer will be a question for you:

"What do you like more: cookies or yourself? What is more important to you: to continue eating those cookies (of which you've already consumed dozens of pounds, and they still taste the same), or to feed your body with good food and keep it healthy?"

My second answer is:

"You WILL eat your favorite cookies if you still want them. You can have some bad food once in a while; it simply will not be your HABIT anymore. When you achieve your ideal weight, feel great, look great and have a new healthy Eating Blueprint, you will THINK and ACT according to that. Based on my experience, you will not be willing to eat those cookies. If you are completely satisfied with your new nutrition style, why would you do something which is not natural to you?"

Here is a simple comparison of two options:

Dieting:

* Many restrictions
* Hunger
* Emotional depression
* Refusing food you love
* Declining social events
* Being back to your habits quickly after the diet is over
* Feelings of guilt that you couldn't keep it
* Gaining even more weight and revoking all your previous efforts

Healthy Eating Lifestyle:

* Changing your habits on the subconscious level
* Replacement vs. declining
* Focusing on your health
* Preventing many diseases
* Right of choice in every situation
* Enjoying social events, cooking and entertaining
* Opportunity to randomly eat "not healthy" food without addiction
* YOU manage the food, the FOOD doesn't manage you

You make your choice. When you change the Eating Blueprint and achieve your ideal weight, your weight trend will stay stable for years, without those "Before" picks and "After" droppings. Making the right choice will become natural, and you'll enjoy it. You'll be surprised how easy it is.

Oh! I almost forgot to mention the 'All inclusive' trips here. Even those won't be difficult for you. Here is what usually happens:

For the first couple of days on an All Inclusive adventure, I automatically choose the food I am used to eating. It's easy, since the choices are many. However, I am not a saint and don't want to be. On day three or so, I start tasting all those cute little sweets, just for curiosity. I can't even say that I enjoy them. Honestly, mostly not. They taste too sweet and too "all the same." But how can you not eat it ALL, if ALL is inclusive? No way! You eat until you blow up! By the time I get home from that crazy feast, I've gained several pounds (in just one week!), and even worse - I don't feel good. Not morally (I admit that I was the only one who did it to myself, and know how to fix it), but physically. My body isn't accustomed to that food, and now suffers. I am so happy to be back to my regular meals, and everything is back to normal in just a week or so. I feel great and promise myself to never-ever go on an All Inclusive trip again (until the next chance I get, I'm afraid...).

Therefore, when your Eating Blueprint is healthy, the goal will be KEEPING your ideal weight. Then, feel free to go for All Inclusive and eat whatever you want. Your body will forgive you that cheating, but please do not take advantage of that. You love your body; so treat it well and feed it with healthy food every day. It will forgive you that act of violence, but not repeatedly. It will not forgive you if you start acting like that too frequently.

I would like to hear your story, so please share it with me. I am pretty confident that your story will be similar to mine, and will confirm the preference of changing the Eating Blueprint over using different diets.

Every process of transformation takes time. Yes, you need to have a goal, make a commitment, unlearn and relearn, uncover the roots and change the Eating Blueprint, Taste your Thoughts and (oh, you bet!) you need to take some action.

Now, I have great news for you: you only do it ONCE! When you do it correctly and passionately, you'll achieve great results and will never have to go through the process again.

Treat your world like a beautiful loveable garden:

❖ Plant good healthy plants (positive and healthy thoughts)

❖ Take good care of the roots (develop new habits, reprogram the existed blueprint)

❖ Invest in future fruits (visualize, use affirmations, declarations, and keep your success journal)

❖ Fight weeds (negative thoughts, your previous habits, wrong believes, and past programming)

❖ Enjoy your gorgeous garden, and be proud of your outstanding outcomes!

"There's only one corner of the Universe you can be certain of improving,

and that's your Own Self."

Aldous Huxley

Declarations:

- *I am proud of all my accomplishments*

- *I live a healthy, joyful, loving life*

- *I am happy, and grateful for every day of my wonderful life*

Chapter 9 : Healthy Feast

"Great cuisine, which is often the simplest cuisine,
has become a recognized art form – an art which, personally,
I would be inclined to place above all others"
Michel Montignac

*L*et's Celebrate! You deserve a feast which will keep you in your desired weight!

3 appetizers + 3 salads + 3 main dishes + 3 desserts!

Cooking is Easy, Quick and Simple!

ᏋᎢᎢᏞᎩ

White Mushrooms with Delicate Cream Cheese-Shrimp Stuffing

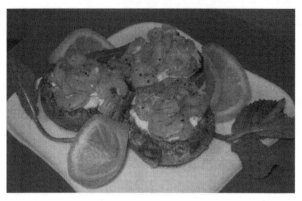

10 medium sized white champignon mushrooms

For stuffing:
½ pound small cocktail shrimps, boiled
1/3 pound of cream cheese
1 teaspoon of lemon juice
1 clove garlic, minced
Fresh ground lemon pepper and nutmeg

Parmesan cheese

Place mushroom cups in a fancy baking dish, sprinkle with salt and pepper.

Mix cream cheese with the lemon juice, garlic and nutmeg. Fill mushroom cups halfway with the cheese mix. Then put several shrimps on top, and sprinkle with lemon pepper and parmesan.

Cook them in a 430*F oven or toaster oven for 10-15 minutes.

ᏬᎢᏛᏬᎩ

Romantic Asparagus

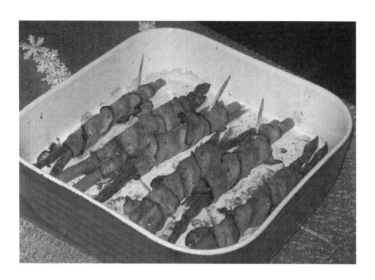

Ingredients:
Fresh asparagus
Smoked meat (low fat bacon, prosciutto, or regular ham)
Flavored olive oil and lemon juice for sprinkling
Fresh ground pepper
Grated Parmesan Cheese

Cut away about one inch of the thick edges of asparagus.

Take 2 spears of asparagus and wrap them with 1 strip of meat. Fix with a wooden toothpick. Put bunches in the baking dish in an opposite directions.

Sprinkle with lemon juice and any flavored olive oil (basil, garlic, rosemary or other). Garnish with fresh ground black pepper and grated Parmesan Cheese.

Please cook the asparagus for 12 minutes <u>exactly</u> (oh, this was finally calculated after many failed experiences) on 450*F in a toaster or regular oven. Serve immediately and enjoy the flavor.

The asparagus may be prepared a night ahead. Cover the baking dish with nylon and keep it in a refrigerator until baking.

The GI of asparagus is very low – only 15. Baked with bacon or prosciutto, it becomes juicier and gets a fantastic flavor. May be consumed with any fresh salad, variety of cold cut meat and cheese. Serve it with a good red wine, and you have a light and delicious romantic dinner.

ᏏᏓᏕᎧ

Fancy Beef Carpaccio

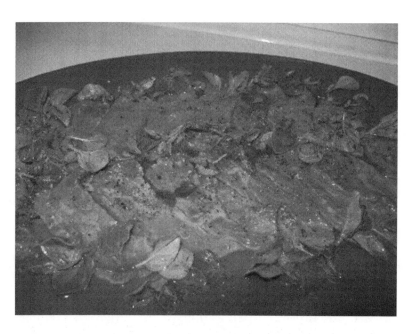

½ pound of beef tenderloin

Vinegar:
5 tablespoons olive oil
Juice of 1 lemon
Salt

On top:
Fresh ground pepper
Fresh oregano leaves (you can use dry oregano too)

Put meat in the freezer for an hour, so it will be cut easier.

Cut into very thin slices and place in one layer in a serving plate.

Mix all the ingredients of the vinegar and pour on the meat. Ground fresh black pepper and arrange oregano leaves on top.

Cover with plastic and put in refrigerator overnight. Great appetizer!

ᢎᠾᡅᠣ

Colorful Green Beans Salad

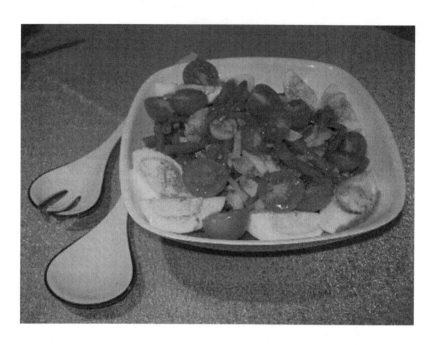

Ingredients:

½ pound frozen green beans, boiled for 2-3 minutes and cooled

2-3 marinated pickles cut into thin 1 inch long strips (please do not replace them with regular salty pickles, the outcome will be different)

¼ of medium size sweet onion, cut into half-rings and rinsed with cold water

1/3 pound smoked turkey ham cut into thin 1 inch long strips

For the top:

2 hardboiled eggs cut into 4 pieces

5-8 cherry tomato cut in halves

Dressing:

1garlic glove

1/3 teaspoon black pepper

½ teaspoon red paprika

¼ teaspoon pure fructose or Splenda

6-7 tablespoons of olive oil

3 tablespoons 5% vinegar

¼ teaspoon kosher salt

½ teaspoon Dijon mustard (do your best to find no sugar mustard)

Gently stir all the ingredients and place into a serving salad dish. Place eggs and cherry tomatoes on top. Mix and slightly bit the dressing ingredients. Pour the dressing over the salad right before serving.

༄

Cozy Fall Avocado Salad

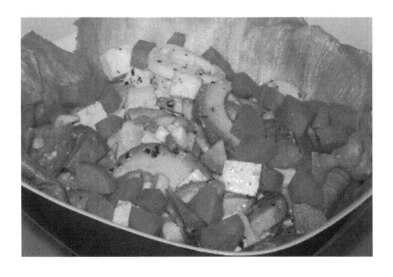

2 avocado
3-4 leaves of green lettuce
1/3 pound white feta cheese
4 boiled hard eggs
Parsley

Dressing:
5 tablespoons of olive oil
1 lemon juice
Salt and fresh ground black pepper

1 carrot

Cut avocado into half, and then cut each half into slices. Cut feta cheese into ½ inch cubes, eggs into 4 pieces and lettuce into medium size flakes. Add parsley, stir gently and place into salad dish.

Mix all the ingredients of the dressing and pour over the salad. Put on the top one carrot, cut into small cubes.

Spring Chickpea Salad

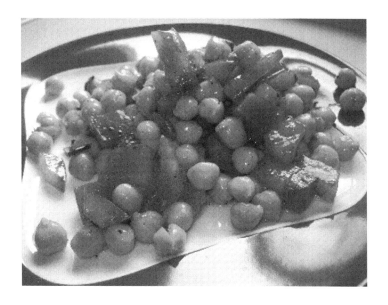

1 can chickpeas
1 big tomato
2 tablespoons of fresh oregano leaves (or basil leaves)
Salt and fresh ground black pepper
Basil flavored olive oil

Cut tomato into small cubes, add all other ingredients and stir gently.

ᏭᎲᎲᏬ

Mediterranean Style Fish Coated with Tomato-Apple Sauce and Feta Cheese

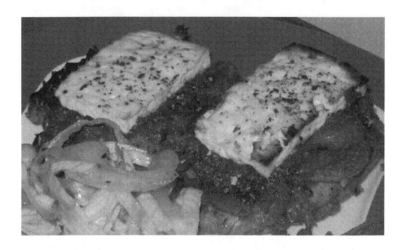

Ingredients:

2 pounds fish of your choice cut into 2x2 inch pieces (use whole if you use small fish fillet)

Sauce:

1 big onion cut into half rings

2 grated Granny Smith apples

2 tablespoons of tomato paste

Salt and fresh ground black pepper

Topping:

½ pound of feta cheese cut into 1x2 inch strips

Thyme if desired

Olive oil for cooking

Cook fish for 2 minutes each side on a thick frying pan on high temperature. Replace it into a baking dish.

In the same pan put the onion and cook until golden-brown. Add tomato paste and grated apples, sprinkle with salt and pepper

Put 1 tablespoon of sauce on each piece of fish, then a strip of cheese on the top. Sprinkle with thyme if you want to.

Cook in a 430*F oven for 20 minutes or until cheese is melted.

Fish may be served by its own, or with fresh salad or wild rice as a side dish.

Chinese Style Meat with Shitake Mushrooms and Vegetables

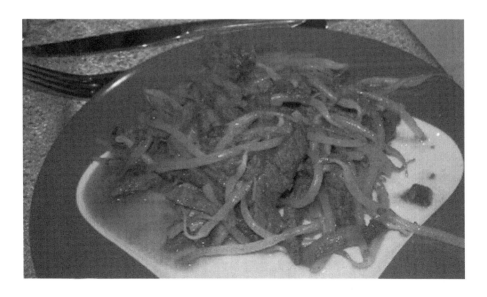

Ingredients:
2 pounds of meat of your choice (chicken breast, pork or beef)
cut into thin about 1 inch long pieces
1 bunch scallions
1 red pepper
2 boxes Shitake mushrooms
1 bag white sprouts

Sauce:
2 tablespoons of mustard (preferably no starch no sugar)
¼ cup of soy sauce
1 tablespoon of sesame oil
1 inch of Ginger root grated
Salt, black pepper and red paprika
Olive oil for cooking.

Preheat a big thick pan, and cook the meat for about 10 minutes, stirring periodically. Meanwhile mix all the ingredients for sauce. When meat is ready, add scallions, red pepper and Shitake. Add sauce, and cook for another 3-5 minutes. At the end add sprouts.

This dish does not require any side dish, but you can add fresh salad, wild rice or whole grain pasta if you wish.

Skinny Mom's Meat Loaf

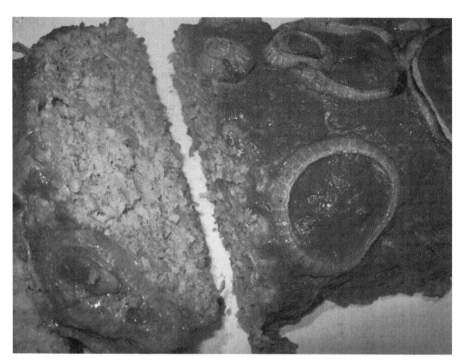

* 1 pound of ground beef
* 1 pound of ground chicken
* 1 pound of ground turkey
* 1 onion, finely chopped
* 1/2 red pepper, chopped
* 2 medium sized white mushrooms, chopped
* ½ cup of whole grain oats
* 1 tablespoon of Worcestershire sauce
* 1 tablespoon of tomato paste or puree
* 2 beaten eggs
* Salt and pepper

2-3 tablespoons of tomato paste and several onion rings for decoration.

Mix well all the ingredients, firm a meatloaf; spread more tomato paste on the top and decorate with onion rings. Cook in 430*F oven for 40-45 minutes.

Please pay attention that there are no bread crumbs in this recipe. They are replaced with much healthier whole grain oats. Oats have a medium Glycemic Index of 40, and totally acceptable. Serve this meat loaf with green salad, fresh vegetables of your choice, boiled green beans or lentils.

ᏩᎥᎡᎢ

Drunken Pears with Sunflower Seeds

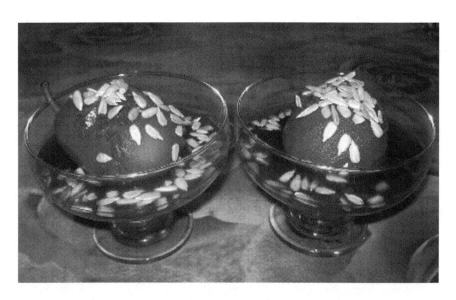

4 green peeled pears
For syrup:
2 cups dry red wine (Merlot or Cabernet)
2 tablespoons of pure fructose or Splenda
1 grated lemon zest
1 cinnamon stick
3-4 whole gloves

Mix all syrup ingredients and bring to boiling. Add pears and boil for another 10 minutes. Put aside for cooling. You can serve them right away, or keep in refrigerator. Sprinkle with sunflower seeds before serving.

ommo

Sweet Memories Apple-Cranberry Cake

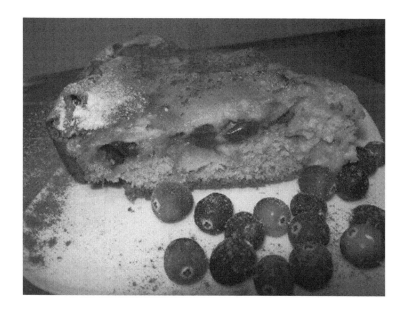

4 big apples of your choice cut into thin lobes
1 cup of fresh or frozen cranberries
1teaspoon of ground cinnamon

Batter mix:
4 eggs
½ cup of Splenda
2/3 cup of oatmeal flour
1/3 cup of sprout flour
1teaspoon of baking powder

Cover round cake pan with a baking paper; arrange layers of apples and cranberries. Sprinkle with ground cinnamon.

Beat eggs with an electric mixer for 2-3 minutes, stir in Splenda and beat another 2 minutes. Add flour and baking powder and stir gently. Pour batter over apples and cranberries.

Bake in 360*F for 35-40 minutes, or until inserted wooden toothpick comes out clean.

Pulling the baking paper remove the cake from the pan, place upside-down on the plate and take out the baking paper.

You can now sprinkle it with more cinnamon, and serve it warm or cold.

Chocolate Mousse

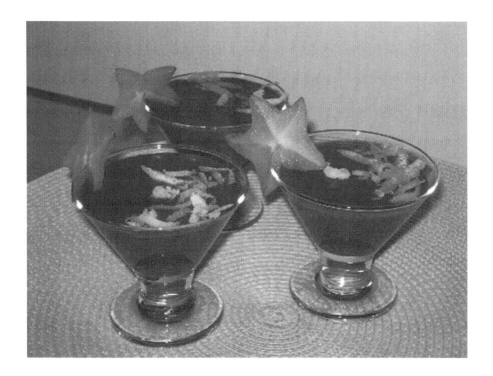

This recipe is a courtesy to Michel Montignac, and the idea is taken from his book "The French GI Diet"

Ingredients:
2 teaspoons of instant coffee
11oz of dark bitter chocolate with 70% cacao
2 fl oz. of Coffee flavored Brandy
1 orange
3 tablespoons of fresh orange juice
6 large eggs

1 pinch of salt

Make a 1/3 cup of strong coffee with the instant coffee.

In a double boiler, melt the chocolate, coffee and brandy. Stir with a wooden spoon until the chocolate has a consistency of a thick, smooth cream. Remove the skillet from the double boiler.

Grate the orange zest, using only the surface part of the peel. Put half the zest in the chocolate mix.

Separate the eggs and put the yolks in a large salad bowl. Whip the whites until stiff. Add 1 pinch of salt at the end and whip again.

Pour the melted chocolate into a salad bowl with the yolks and mix well. Add the whites gradually and stir gently.

Fill individual dessert dishes, sprinkle with the rest of the orange zest and chill for at least 6 hours.

The GI of chocolate which contains more than 70% cacao is only 20. The recipe does not include bad carbs or saturated fats. Enjoy it and get slim!

"The best diet is the one you don't know you are on"
Brian Wansink, Ph.D.

Appendix

Glycemic Index Table

HIGH GI

Corn syrup	115
Beer*	110
Glucose (dextrose)	100
Glucose syrup	100
Modified starch	100
Wheat syrup, rice syrup	100
Maltodextrin	95
Potato flour (starch)	95
Potatoes fried, french fries, scalloped potatoes	95
Potatoes, oven cooked	95
Rice flour	95
Bread white Gluten-free	90
Potato flour	90
Rice sticky	90
Arrow-root	85

Carrots (cooked)*	85
Celeriac, knob celery, turnip rooted celery (cooked)*	85
Corn flakes	85
Hamburger buns	85
Instant/parboiled rice	85
Maizena (corn starch)	85
Parsnip*	85
Pop corn (without sugar)	85
Rice cake/pudding	85
Rice Crispies	85
Rice milk	85
Tapioca	85
Turnip (coked)*	85
White sandwich bread	85
White wheat flour	85
Kellogg's Cornflakes	84
Pretzels	83
Kellogg's Rice Krispies	82
Jelly Beans	80
Mashed potatoes	80
Chips	75
Corn cooked	75
Doughnuts	75
Grahams Crackers	75
Lasagna (soft wheat)	75
Pumpkin, gourd*	75
Squash/marrow (various)*	75
Waffle (with sugar)	75
Watermelon*	75
Corn chips	74

Kavli Crispbread	71
Bagels	70
Baguette white bread	70
Biscuit	70
Brioche	70
Cabbage turnip, rutabaga, Swede turnip	70
Chocolate bar (with sugar added)	70
Cola drinks, soft drinks, sodas	70
Corn flour	70
Croissant	70
Dates Dried	70
Gnocchi	70
Matzo bread (white flour)	70
Millet, sorghum	70
Molasses	70
Noodles (tender wheat)	70
Pealed boiled potatoes	70
Plantain/cooking banana/platano (cooked)	70
Polenta, cornmeal	70
Potato boiled	70
Potato chips, crisps	70
Potato, tinned	70
Puffed amaranth	70
Ravioli (soft wheat)	70
Refined cereals (with sugar added)	70
Rice bread	70
Risotto	70
Rusk	70
Special K™	70
Rice standard	70

Tacos	70
White sugar (sucrose)	70
Whole brown sugar	70
Cake, angel	67
Green pea soup, tinned	66
Beans Fava, broad bean, horse bean (cooked)	65
Beet, beetroot (cooked)*	65
Bread Rye flour (30% of rye)	65
Cake, tart	65
Cantaloupe	65
Chestnut flour	65
Chinese noodles/vermicelli (rice)	65
Couscous, semolina	65
Cranberry dried (sugar added)	65
Hovis, brown bread (with leaven)	65
Jam (with sugar added)	65
Macaroni cheese	65
Maple syrup	65
Marmalade (with sugar)	65
Mars®, Sneakers®, Nuts®, etc. bars	65
Muesli (with sugar or honey added...)	65
Muffin Blueberry	65
Panapen, breadfruit, breadnut	65
Pineapple (tin/can)	65
Potato Unpeeled boiled/steamed	65
Quince (preserve/jelly, with sugar)	65
Raisins (red and golden)	65
Sorbet (with sugar added)	65
Spelt, einkorn	65
Sushi	65

Corn, sweet corn	65
Tamarind, Indian date (sweet)	65
Tropical yam -US-, yam	65
Whole-grain bread	65
Apricots (tin/can with syrup)	64
Bean black soup,tinned	64
Bananas	60
Barley Pearl	60
Bread Pita	60
Chestnut	60
Danish pastry	60
Hard/durum wheat semolina	60
Honey	60
Ice cream (regular, with sugar added)	60
Lasagna (hard wheat)	60
Long-grain white rice	60
Mayonnaise (industrial, sweetened)	60
Melons (cantaloupe, honeydew, etc.)*	60
Milk loaf, milk white	60
Muffin unsweetened	60
Rice Perfumed (jasmine...)	60
Pizza	60
Chocolate powder (with sugar)	60
Ravioli (hard wheat)	60
Bulgur wheat (cooked)	55
Butter cookies, shortbread, spritz biscuit (flour, butter, sugar)	55
Grape juice (unsweetened)	55
Japanese plum, loquat	55
Kellogg's Special K	55
Ketchup	55

Mango juice (unsweetened)	55
Mustard (sugar added)	55
Nutella®	55
Oatmeal Cookies	55
Papaya (fresh fruit)	55
Peaches (tin/can, with syrup)	55
Red rice	55
Spaghetti (well cooked)	55
Tagliatelle (well cooked)	55
Crisps	54
Lentils Green, tinned	52
Kellogg's All Bran	51

MEDIUM GI

Apple juice (unsweetened)	50
Barley, whole grain	50
Biscuit (whole flour, no sugar added)	50
Bread multi grain	50
Bread with quinoa (approximately 65% of quinoa)	50
Cereal bar, energetic (no sugar added)	50
Chayote, chocho, pear squash, christophine	50
Cranberry juice (unsweetened)	50
Kiwi fruit	50
Linguine	50
Litchi (fresh fruit)	50
Macaroni (durum wheat)	50
Mango (fresh fruit)	50
Muesli (no sweet)	50
Persimmon, kaki-persimmon	50

Pineapple juice (unsweetened)	50
Potatoes Sweet	50
Rice Basmati	50
Rice Brown, unpolished rice	50
Tomato soup, tinned	50
Wasa™ light rye	50
Whole wheat pasta	50
Beans baked, tinned	48
Bread Rye (integral; flour, bread)	45
Coconut	45
Cranberry	45
Farro flour (integral)	45
Grapefruit juice (unsweetened)	45
Grapes, green and red (fresh fruit)	45
Green peas (tin/can)	45
Jam (no sugar added, grapefruit juice sweetened)	45
Kamut bread	45
Kamut flour (integral)	45
Kellogg's Bran Buds	45
Orange juice (fresh squeezed and unsweetened)	45
Pineapple (fresh fruit)	45
Plantain/cooking banana/platano (raw)	45
Plantain/cooking banana/platano (raw)	45
Rice Brown Basmati	45
Spelt, einkorn (integral)	45
Spelt, einkorn (integral)	45
Tomato sauce (with sugar)	45
Whole bulgur wheat (cooked)	45
Whole cereals (no sugar added)	45
Whole couscous, whole semolina	45

Lentil soup, tinned	44
Beans Black-eyed	41
Beans Fava, broad beans, horse beans (raw)	40
Bread, 100% integral flour with pure leaven	40
Brut cider	40
Buckwheat, kasha (grain or flour)	40
Carrot juice (unsweetened)	40
Coconut milk	40
Egyptian wheat, kamut	40
Falafel (fava beans)	40
Farro	40
Fig Dried	40
Integral wheat pasta, al dente	40
Beans Kidney/pinto (tin/can)	40
Lactose	40
Matzo bread (integral flour)	40
Oats	40
Peanut butter (no suger addes)	40
Pepino dulce, melon pear	40
Plums Dried /prunes	40
Quince (preserve/jelly, without sugar)	40
Quinoa flour	40
Shortbread, spritz biscuit (integral flour, no sugar added)	40
Sorbet (unsweetened)	40
Spagetti whole wheat	40
Spaghetti 'Al dente' (5 min cook)	40
Tahin	40

LOW GI

Apple (fresh fruit)	35
Apple stew, apple sauce	35
Apples (dried)	35
Beans Black	35
Beans Chick Peas, garbanzo beans (tin/can)	35
Bread Essene/ezekiel (sprouted cereals bread)	35
Celeriac, knob celery, turnip rooted celery (raw)	35
Chick pea flour	35
Chinese noodles/vermicelli (hard wheat), noodles	35
Bean Cranberry, borlotti bean, Roman bean	35
Dijon type mustard	35
Falafel (chick peas)	35
Figs; Indian/barbary fig (fresh fruit)	35
Green peas (fresh)	35
Ice cream (with real fructose)	35
Indian corn	35
Beans Kidney/pinto	35
Linum, sesame (seeds)	35
Nectarines (fresh fruit)	35
Oranges (fresh fruit)	35
Peaches (fresh fruit)	35
Plums, prunes (fresh fruit)	35
Pomegranate (fresh fruit)	35
Quince (fresh fruit)	35
Quinoa, hie	35
Rice Wild	35
Soy yogurt (fruit flavored)	35
Sunflower seeds	35

Tomato juice	35
Tomato sauce (natural, no sugar added)	35
Tomatos Dried	35
Wasa™ fiber (24%)	35
White almond paste/puree (unsweetened)	35
Yeast	35
Yogurt**	35
Beans Cannellini	31
Almond milk	30
Apricots (dried)	30
Apricots (fresh fruit)	30
Beans Chick Peas, garbanzo	30
Beans French, string beans	30
Beans Red Kidney	30
Beet (raw)	30
Carrots (raw)	30
Chinese noodles/vermicelli (made from soy or mung beans)	30
Garlic	30
Grapefruit, pummelo, shaddock (fresh fruit)	30
Lentils	30
Lentils Brown	30
Lentils Yellow	30
Marmalade (no sugar added)	30
Milk** (skimmed or not)	30
Oat milk (non cooked)	30
Passion fruit, maracuja, granadilla	30
Pears (fresh fruit)	30
Milk powdered/fresh **	30
Quark, curd cheese**	30
Soya milk	30
Tangerines, madarines, satsuma	30

Tomatoes	30
Turnip (raw)	30
Lentils Green, boiled	29
Barley Blanched	25
Blackberry, mulberry	25
Blueberry, whortleberry, bilberry	25
Cherries	25
Dark chocolate (more than 70% of cocoa content)	25
Gooseberry	25
Hummus	25
Beans Mung , moong dal	25
Peanut paste/puree (unsweetened)	25
Raspberry (fresh fruit)	25
Redcurrant	25
Seeds (squash/marrow)	25
Soy flour	25
Split peas	25
Strawberries (fresh fruit)	25
Whole-hazelnut paste/puree (unsweetened)	25
Artichoke	20
Bamboo shoot	20
Chocolate, plain (>85% of cocoa)	20
Eggplant	20
Fructose	20
Heart of palm, cabbage palm	20
Lemon	20
Lemon juice (unsweetened)	20
Cocoa powder (no sugar added)	20
Ratatouille	20
Soy \"cream\"	20
Soy yogurt (unflavored)	20

Tamari sauce (unsweetened)	20
West Indian cherry, acerola	20
Soybeans	16
Agave (syrup)	15
Almonds	15
Asparagus	15
Black currant	15
Bran (oat, wheat...)	15
Broccoli	15
Brussels sprouts	15
Cabbage	15
Carob powder	15
Cashew nut, acajou	15
Cauliflower	15
Celery	15
Cereal shoots (soy or mung bean sprouts, etc.)	15
Chicory, endive	15
Chili pepper	15
Courgettes, zucchini	15
Cucumber	15
Fennel	15
Ginger	15
Golden gooseberry, Cape gooseberry	15
Green beans	15
Hazelnuts, filberts, Barcelona nuts	15
Leeks, scallions	15
Lettuce, all varieties	15
Mushroom, fungus	15
Olives	15
Onions	15
Peanuts	15

Pesto	15
Pickle	15
Pine seed	15
Pistachio, green almond	15
Radish	15
Rhubarb	15
Runner beans, Italian flat beans	15
Sauerkraut, sourcrout	15
Shallot, echalot, Spanish garlic	15
Snow peas	15
Sorrel dock	15
Soya	15
Spinach beet, perpetual spinach	15
Spinaches	15
Sprouted seeds	15
Peppers sweet (red, green), paprika	15
Tempeh	15
Tofu, soybean curd	15
Walnuts	15
Wheat germ	15
Avocado	10
Crustaceans	5
Spices (parsley, basil, oregano, cinnamon, vanilla, etc.)	5
Vinegar	5

* These products have high GI, but their pure sugar content (pure glucid) is low (about 5%). Therefore they should not significantly affect blood sugar levels.

** There is no difference in the GI of whole-milk products and non-fat milk products, however they have high Insulinic Index.

Benefit from other products and services offered by Dr. IRINA

www.WeightDestiny.com

FREE 5 day email-course "Top 10 Tips to Achieve Your Goal of Reducing Weight"

Brochure: '10 Mushrooms Recipes for Your Romantic Dinner'

Easy downloadable full color brochure provides you with recipes for delicious and easy-to-make meals. They can be served as appetizers or as a main dish.

Positive Affirmation MP3 files: *Ideal Weight and Super Self*

Easy downloadable files provide you with positive affirmations, which are short motivational sentences with motivational music in the background. Sentences are in the present tense, so they can be absorbed better by your subconscious mind. There is a pause after each sentence where you need to repeat that sentence out loud and visualize your desired image. You can listen to it anytime anywhere. The more frequently you listen, repeat and FEEL your desire, the better it is absorbed subconsciously. Which means you will achieve your goals quicker and easier.

Personal Coaching:

You get what you truly want much faster and easier when you have your own personal coach and mentor who walks you through the process focusing on your individual needs.

* Uncover hidden causes of your being overweight and improve your eating habits forever

* Discover healthy nutrition tips matching your individual needs

* Enhance your inner peace and happiness, as well as self image

Cooking and Coaching classes

Perfect for a girls' party or entertaining friends. 3 hours of Weight Loss and LIFE Coaching in your place. You get weight loss coaching tips and new recipes. You cook, eat, laugh and have fun with your friends!

* We create a menu for lunch or dinner according to your preferences

* Together we cook the entire lunch/dinner, from appetizer to dessert, with your 6-10 friends/ family at your home

* You discover how easily you can adjust your favorite recipes, and to apply Low GI nutrition to everyday life

Weight Loss Coaching Program: CHOOSE YOUR WEIGHT

You will walk out of the program with an entirely brand-new knowledge, skills and habits, and outlook on yourself, your health and your whole life!

* Step-by-step process how to permanently change your Eating Habits Blueprint

* Use powerful mind-setting tools and exercises, weight loss imagery and declarations

* Understand food categories and principles of low GI nutrition to enjoy a gourmet food and stay slim and healthy forever

* Share experience, challenges and achievements with new likeminded friends and have fun!

Use your book receipt number and get FREE BONUSES

$50 off your first month of Private Coaching

$50 off your group Cooking and Coaching Classes

$50 off your Weight Loss Coaching Program: CHOOSE YOUR WEIGHT

Connect with Dr. IRINA online:

www.WeightDestiny.com
www.Journey2Destiny.com
www.TasteOfThoughts.com

Facebook @Weight Loss Program
Twitter @ WeightDestiny
LinkedIN @ Dr. Irina Koles

Together, we'll make YOUR dreams a reality!

To your Health and Success

Dr. Irina

Made in the USA
Charleston, SC
10 May 2012